Never Diet Again!

Learn the secrets to a lean and fit body without dieting

BETTERBODY BETTERLIFE

Croix Sather

Ken,
Find the possibility
in the problems!
Get past the challenges
in your mind and
anything is possible!
with appreciation
and love,
Croix

ReneCruz LLC

Renato Publishing
A company of ReneCruz LLC.
RenatoPublishing.com

rp
RENATO
PUBLISHING

THE BETTERBODY BETTERLIFE PROGRAM IS INTENDED FOR HEALTHY ADULTS, AGE 18 AND OVER. THIS BOOK IS SOLELY FOR INFORMATIONAL AND EDUCATIONAL PURPOSES AND IS NOT MEDICAL ADVICE. THE AUTHOR IS NOT A PHYSICIAN AND THE IDEAS, PROCEDURES, AND SUGGESTIONS IN THIS BOOK ARE NOT A SUBSTITUTE FOR SEEKING MEDICAL ADVICE. PLEASE CONSULT A MEDICAL OR HEALTH PROFESSIONAL BEFORE YOU BEGIN ANY NEW EXERCISE OR NUTRITION PROGRAM, OR IF YOU HAVE QUESTIONS ABOUT YOUR HEALTH. THIS BOOK REPRESENTS WHAT CAN BE ACCOMPLISHED THROUGH AN INTEGRATED SYSTEM OF EXERCISE, NUTRITION, AND PLANNING. AS INDIVIDUALS DIFFER, THEIR RESULTS WILL DIFFER, EVEN WHEN USING THE SAME PROGRAM.

FIRST EDITION

Library of Congress Cataloging-in-Publications Data

Sather, Croix

BetterBody BetterLife: Connecting the Mind with the Body for Permanent Weight Loss Without Dieting/Croix Sather.- 1st ed.

ISBN-13: 978-0-9746178-0-0 LCCN: 2003098319

1. Weight loss 2. Exercise. 3. Physical fitness. 4. Health. I. Title.

Visit us on the web: BETTERBODYBETTERLIFE.COM
RENATOPUBLISHING.COM RENECRUZ.COM

Renato Publishing books may be purchased for educational, business, or sales promotional use. For information, please write: Special Markets Department, Renato Publishing, PO Box 8834, New Fairfield, CT 06812 or contact via email at OrderServices@RenatoPublishing.com

From the back cover: † FTC Red Flag; Bogus Weight Loss Claims http://www.ftc.gov/redflag

Cover by: Tabitha Pearson Marshall
Editing: Faith Brynie; and Pnuema Books

Also by Croix Sather

BetterBody BetterLife program
BetterBody BetterLife audio book
BetterBody BetterLife Fitness DVD
BetterBody BetterLife Journal
BetterBody BetterLife Picture Plaque
BetterBody BetterLife Exercise Posters
BetterBody BetterLife videos

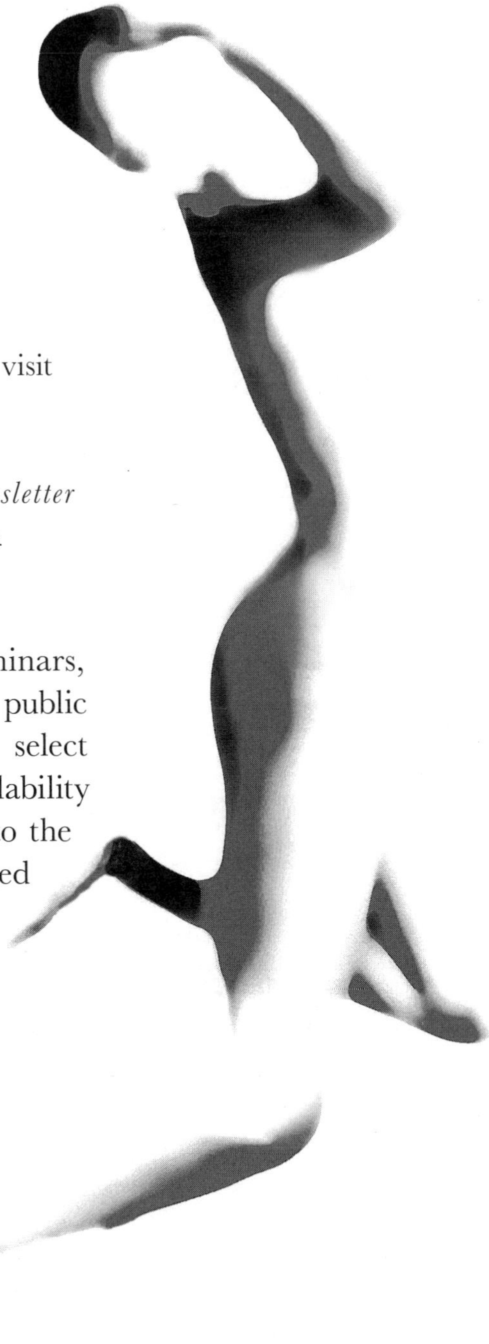

For more information and to order please visit
www.BetterBodyBetterLife.com

Get the FREE *BetterBody BetterLife Newsletter*
visit **www.BetterBodyBetterLife.com**
Click on ***Newsletter*** to get more free.

Croix Sather is available for seminars, keynote speeches, workshops, and public events. He provides consulting for select clients. Requests, inquiries, and availability for these services should be directed to the address below. Readers are encouraged to contact the author with comments about this book and ideas or recommendations for future editions.

BetterBody BetterLife
Attention: Public Appearances
PO Box 8834
New Fairfield, CT 06812

email: seminars@BetterBodyBetterLife.com
or: mainbox@BetterBodyBetterLife.com
or visit: www.BetterBodyBetterLife.com

Never Diet Again!

Learn the secrets to a lean and fit body without dieting

BETTERBODY BETTERLIFE

Croix Sather

This book is dedicated to those who are looking for the inner power to change their lives.

APPRECIATION

BetterBody BetterLife became possible with the help of some very special people. First I want to thank my wife, Tina, who has taught me so much with so few words. Her enduring patience and endless love have been my guide and motivation. My children have taught me a new level of love. Many influence us, and my family has had a great influence on me — especially my mom, who is proof that a woman can be feminine, loving, and powerful; and my dad who provided me with a great foundation to succeed in life including an entrepreneurial spirit, and taught me that great achievements can come at every stage in life.

I am grateful to my wonderful and treasured friend Jean Flynn, who helped me get this book off and running, and has been an amazing friend. I also thank my confidants and advisors, Dave "The Wheel" Wheeler, Rob Ferrucci, Michael and Mary Beth, Alex and Amy, and Randy Bogues. Thanks also to my sports buddies for keeping me on my game and making fitness fun.

Special thanks for their invaluable help and professional advice on this book to Doug Mateo; Faith Brynie, my exceptional editor; Nina Taylor of Pneuma Books; Tab Pearson Marshall for an amazing book cover design; Karen Raftery Photography; AXA Media Group; and Anita Fabian. Your expertise has been astonishing.

And special mention to my sister Rachel and brothers Ray and Darrin; Jose Salgado, Jefferson Wiggins, Peggy Katkocin, Ed Tate, Marilyn, Chuck, and my Toastmasters friends. Thank you all for being wonderful people to emulate and catalysts of change in my life.

Words cannot truly express my appreciation. *Thank you all.*

About the Author

Hello Friends,

I remember keeping my brother company in the basement when he "pumped iron." In that cold, damp room, my child's mind dreamed of becoming strong and muscular like a superhero. Fitness became a passion, and I devoured every bodybuilding magazine and book written by the fitness icons of that era. This was during the incredible growth stage of the fitness industry in the 1980s, only a few years after Arnold Schwarzenegger won his seventh Mr. Olympia title and during the time when Cory Everson won the Ms. Olympia six years in a row. The world of fitness and bodybuilding left a lasting impression that endures with me today.

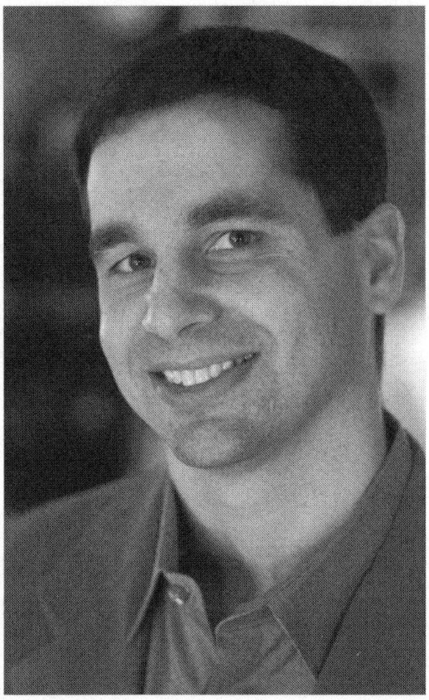

I spent my teenage and college years in the gym aspiring to become a professional bodybuilder. Then life started. As the years passed, work replaced gym time, and family and friends filled spare time. Like most people, my crammed schedule left no time for exercise, and my fast-paced life with even faster meals promoted the growth of a spare tire. Although I knew how to keep fit and lean, the "speed of life" got in the way — as it does for many of us. That is until I decided I had had enough. Getting fat and out of shape, I decided to take back my life and find the best way to create a ***better body*** and a ***better life***.

I went back to school to study social sciences. I wanted to understand why people do what they do, even when their actions sometimes create pain. I researched fitness, nutrition, personal development, neurolinguistic programming, meditation, communication, the psychology of weight loss, and the psychology of success. My certification as a holistic fitness practitioner with the National Exercise and Sports Trainers Association attests to my knowledge of personal training, cardiovascular exercise, mental skills development, and yoga. I never stop learning. I continue to build on current knowledge and explore new areas of study from our culture and abroad. I believe that if you are not growing, you are dying. Growth comes from learning, believing, achieving, sharing, and contributing.

I know there is more to weight loss than just mechanics and logistics. With over 65 percent of Americans overweight, there has to be a better method for shedding body fat than diets, pills, and surgery. The result of my work is the *BetterBody BetterLife* plan. This plan is the reason that I am in better health and shape now than I was twenty years ago. You can be, too!

I want to help you become the person you have always dreamed of being. I see so much pain in the lives of people. Much of their pain can be avoided or dramatically reduced if they live a healthy lifestyle. I want to help you free yourself from the prison that years of neglect and misinformation have caused. My life is filled with excitement and jubilation because I have found these secrets to a full and balanced life and because I have the opportunity to share them with you.

LIVE FIT, WORK HARD, PLAY HARDER, LAUGH OFTEN, LOVE MOST.

LIFE IS A WONDERFUL RIDE!

All the best,

Table of Contents

Main Sections

Chapters

We are each responsible for our own life -
no other person is or even can be.

Oprah Winfrey

Foreword

By Dr. Doug Mateo

We attempt to maintain balance in all aspects of our complex lives. At times events derail our efforts and create an imbalance. Whether the imbalance is internal (our mind and body) or external (home and work), balance must be regained for proper functioning. When patients come to me for chiropractic treatment, I often see a partial or complete loss of balance in their lives and bodies. The imbalance manifests itself as pain, spasms, obesity, muscular atrophy, or mental and physical fatigue.

Modern life can disrupt the balance by tempting us with fast food, unhealthy routines, overscheduling, and self-abuse...all of which elevate stress. Most of us have a profound lack of knowledge about what our bodies require to function properly, so we find ourselves out of balance and susceptible to ill health — sometimes even creating all sorts of illnesses.

Croix has a wonderful approach to helping ordinary people achieve balance in their lives. His methods help individuals recognize interferences in their lives that accelerate the loss of balance. The best way to regain balance, reduce illness, and avoid injuries is to lose excess body fat and maintain a healthy weight.

From this book, you will learn that even little changes can make a big difference. Here Croix provides guidance on setting goals and suggests multiple ways to achieve those goals. His book provides appropriate exercises, muscle-toning routines, and a dietary plan that is consistent with his wonderful philosophy. All of the approaches that *BetterBody BetterLife* teaches can help you earn a healthy, stable quality of life, eliminate imbalances, and live at a healthy weight. Take the first step today for a new balance tomorrow.

*Doug Mateo is a physician of chiropractic care formerly in New York, and now practicing at Mateo Chiropractic in Eudora, Kansas.

Is This Book for You?

You've tried diet after diet without success. Like a yo-yo, your weight goes up and down and then up even higher. If you want to stop dieting and start living, then this book is for you. Living at a healthy weight without dieting occurs only when you make health a foundation of your life. The *BetterBody BetterLife Plan* is a lifestyle change. No gimmicks and literally no bologna!

This book is for those who want to live a life without dieting, pills, shakes, meetings, or surgery. It is for those who are ready to take control of their lives and who want to live life to its fullest but still eat real food. It's for those who want to enjoy time with friends and family without worrying about eating too much or too little protein, too many or too few carbohydrates.

In this book, you will learn to live the way you were built to live. You will learn to make healthy choices, and you will learn when it's okay not to. You will learn to live an active, full life. This approach may be different from the life you are living now, but your present habits may have you on the road to heart-attack city. Worse, you may be trapped in a living purgatory as a sedentary, obese individual who watches life go by without being able to participate. That description may sound gloomy, but so is that kind of life.

A Healthy Lifestyle

A healthy lifestyle is a mainstream event, so mainstream that you no longer need to go to a small health food market to find unprocessed food. Most supermarkets have a "health" or "natural" foods section, and health food supermarkets are popping up around globe. The leading health food supermarket has nearly 200 stores in North America and the United Kingdom.

A healthy lifestyle is supported by time-honored traditions, cultures from around the world, the latest research, and even tree-hugging, granola-eating extremists. Because of our global economy and instant, worldwide communications, we have immediate access to almost any food and almost any kind of information. We can often bypass information gatekeepers and get untainted information directly from the source. This gives the ordinary person an unprecedented opportunity to make informed choices.

About the Content

Deciding how much information was the right amount for this book was difficult. I realize that you have a busy life and you probably do not want to read a 600-page fitness book. However, you need a certain amount of information to live without dieting and to succeed at managing your weight and fitness.

BetterBody BetterLife is divided into three sections: "Building Your Foundation," "Nourishing Nutrition," and "Fitness for a Fabulous Body." The information in these three sections works in synergy to make a life without dieting possible. Neglect any one of them and your odds of success are miniscule. This three-section division makes referring back to specific information easier. In addition to this book is a DVD to show you how to perform the muscle-toning exercises properly and comfortably.

The information you are about to read is critical in your learning process. It is nearly timeless; it will be just as valid 5, 10, or even 20 years from now as it is today. Of course the scientific world will discover some new information, but the *BetterBody BetterLife* plan is about learning the physiological fundamentals of the human body. That is the foundation you can build your life on.

How to Use This Book

You can read this book from the first page to the last, but you do not have to. If you already have some exercise knowledge or you are eager to get started in the program, you may choose to preview the "Fitness for a Fabulous Body" section first. If you do, you can start some exercises while you are reading the rest of the book. The body requires a slow and deliberate beginning pace to avoid excessive soreness and to minimize the chances of injury. However, a slow pace in starting to exercise is not lost time. It is the beginning of your transformation to the splendor of fit living, a healthy lifestyle, and a great physique.

Keep this book for future reference. There are many sections that will prove useful over time. As it is said, "Repetition is the mother of all skills."

THE PAST DOES **NOT** EQUAL THE FUTURE.
IT IS UP TO YOU TO **CREATE** YOUR FUTURE.

How to Take Control of Your Life

It seems to happen overnight. One day you wake up, look in the mirror, and ask, 'When did I get so fat?" The speed of life pushes many important things to the wayside.

When you ignore your health and fitness, fat slowly fills the voids in your body and eventually pushes outward, distorting your physique. You are fat because you intentionally or unintentionally neglected your dietary intake and your fitness plan. You may not have enough information or accurate information. You may be self-sabotaging, or you may not have the motivation or leverage to create lasting results.

IT IS TIME FOR A CHANGE.

You must take responsibility for your life, your actions, and reactions. If you are looking for a plan that will tell you it's not your fault you are overweight, or if you are looking for a plan that will make you thin while sitting in your recliner, then go find a different book. I empathize with you, and I want to help you, but I will not lie to you. Anyone who promises results without your participation is deceiving you. The only way that you will get what you want out of life is to take possession of your destiny. Your past may have influenced who you are, but you are responsible for who you become. To get past the challenge of being overweight, you and you alone must make changes.

PERMANENT WEIGHT LOSS WITHOUT DIETING.

This book is about much more than how to shed weight. Losing weight, or more accurately losing body fat, is simply a by-product of the *BetterBody BetterLife* plan. A healthy life at a fit weight without dieting is the focus of this plan. When you empower yourself with knowledge and find the motivation that generates the right choices, you will become healthy and fit. In this process, you will lose body fat, take inches off your waist, trim your thighs, and sculpt a beautiful work of art.

Health and fitness are much more than eating right and exercising. They involve making a commitment to yourself, loving yourself, and refusing to accept anything less than a great life. The *BetterBody BetterLife* plan is a healthful way of living based on logic, balance, and time-honored knowledge, as well as the latest information. You will find some information goes against the mainstream beliefs. Bureaucratic processes, political pressure, and irresponsible oversight taint much of the information promoted by government organizations. In an effort to make quick megaprofits, pharmaceutical companies, corporations, and savvy marketing professionals inundate society with gadgets and quick fix gimmicks. But don't worry! The side effects are only life threatening. Where does this leave us? Question everything and take ownership of your fate.

I have good news for you. If you are not willing to take responsibility for your actions, then there is no reason for you to read any further. If you choose not to be the master of your life and destiny, then go ahead and put this book down.

I am happy that you are still reading because your life is about to change. Between here and the back cover is the information you need to become fit and healthy, lose body fat, and get more out of life – all without dieting and in less than 3 percent of your day.

You have only one chance at life.

Make it worth the ride!

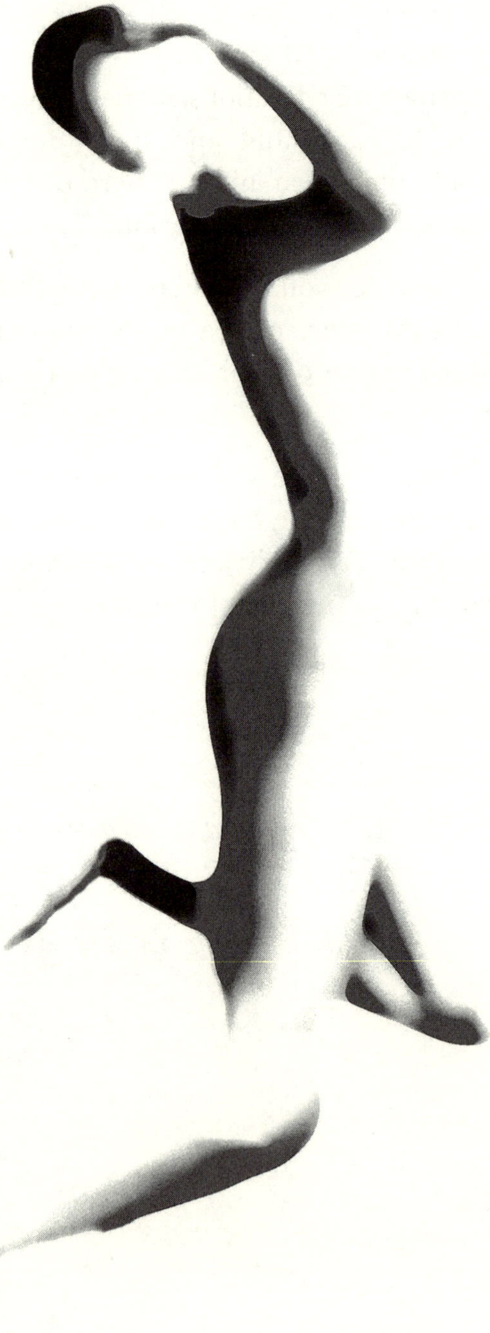

Section One

Building Your Foundation

Chapter One

WHAT TO EXPECT

How many people do you know who are dieting right now? How many kinds of diets have you heard of? How many have you tried? With so many diets, why do so many people fail at losing weight, staying fit, and keeping healthy?

THE REASON IS THIS: DIETS DON'T WORK!

Yes, it is true. Diets do not work! Everyday we are inundated with the latest, greatest, surefire, guaranteed miracle diet. Diets are fads and scams. They confuse us and promote the yo-yo effect, temporary weight loss followed by an inevitable regain and more. There are many diet plans to choose from; with most of them, you are doomed to fail before you even begin. Diets are not the answer.

The results attained through dieting are rarely permanent or effective because "diets" are not meant to be a permanent solution. The contemporary definition of the word [to] "diet" is to cause sudden weight loss in a short amount of time. When the "dieting" stops and the previous eating habits resume, the weight comes back with a vengeance and weight goes up; hence the yo-yo effect. Don't confuse the contemporary term [to] "diet" with one's personal diet. Everyone has a diet or dietary intake. One's diet may be healthful, balanced, good, bad, dreadful, or worse, whether he or she is "on a diet" or not.

Why is this plan different? This is not a diet! The *BetterBody BetterLife* plan is healthy living through a balanced lifestyle. I believe that 97 percent of weight loss is between your ears. Where your mind goes, your body will follow.

In only 30 minutes a day, you can have the body that you have always dreamed about. You can lose weight and become fit. In this book, you will learn my *Trilogy of Health* approach to successful, permanent weight loss, weight management, and fitness. From start to finish, this book will guide you to your goals. *BetterBody BetterLife* is a step-by-step plan that leaves nothing in question.

WHAT'S AHEAD?

There are no quick miracles when it comes to permanent weight loss and healthy living. However, the path to both can be simple and straightforward. A healthy life requires knowledge, energy, and most important, a desire to change. When I started my research, I looked for shortcuts to healthy living and weight loss because, like you, I don't want to take any more time or energy to be healthy than is required. I've found that there are no shortcuts to weight loss and a healthy body. In my countless hours of research and planning, I have simplified the only true recipe for success. It is the way I live and the way many people live who have achieved a long-term healthy lifestyle. This plan is not a secret. It is the proven and permanent way to lose weight and live healthily…made easy. I will not lead you to believe that the plan does not require effort. It does. There are no gimmicks here. However, this book distills a mountain of information into a few simple-to-follow steps so you can achieve your weight loss dreams.

Compared to the endless rollercoaster of "being on a diet" with the loss and inevitable regain of body fat and compared to living in a state of overweight or obesity, this plan is easy. Very easy! In the *BetterBody BetterLife* plan, you will find everything you need to be successful in your journey toward a richer life through healthy living.

Let's take a look at what will happen for you with this plan… and what won't.

YOU WILL NOT:

You will NOT spend hours a day exercising.
You will NOT have to join a gym.
You will NOT have to become a health "guru."
You will NOT be on a high-protein or a low-carbohydrate diet.
You will NOT be on any diet.
You will NOT have to give up your favorite foods.
You will NOT skip meals or starve yourself.
You will NOT have to weigh any of your food.
You will NOT be hungry.
There are no shakes or protein bars.
There are no pills.
There are no meals to buy.
There are no meetings to attend.
There are no gadgets.
There are no gimmicks.

YOU WILL:

YOU WILL be able to lose weight and keep it off.
YOU WILL have more energy and strength.
YOU WILL enjoy what you see in the mirror.
YOU WILL feel great about who you are.
YOU WILL be able to buy clothes in any retail store.
YOU WILL enjoy your life to the fullest.
YOU WILL have more confidence.
YOU WILL have a better attitude.
YOU WILL have less stress.
YOU WILL be able to have snacks.
YOU WILL eat full and satisfying meals.
YOU WILL be able to enjoy all of your favorite foods.
YOU WILL have a diverse menu.
YOU WILL have a better quality of life.
YOU WILL live guilt free.

You will NOT feel guilty! You will not live on beans and wheat, coconuts, cabbage soup, or grapefruits, nor will you spend your entire day exercising. You will have a wonderfully diverse and satisfying menu, probably even more than you do now. Living well does not require more work. In fact, it is less work and less stressful. It provides infinite rewards.

Imagine

Imagine a life in which you wake up in the morning and love what you see in the mirror. You don't have to worry about an outfit making you look fat, and you head out the door with a rhythm in your step. You have enough energy to propel you through the day and enough energy for your family and friends after work. Imagine a life where you are not self-conscious about your body. You walk on the beach in a swimsuit and feel good! At night, you don't want to turn the lights off in the bedroom or keep a robe within inches of your bed.

You're Not Alone

Living a healthy life at a healthy weight evades over two-thirds of Americans. Sixty-five percent of Americans range from being overweight to obese according to the 1999-2002 National Health and Nutrition Examination Survey (NHANES). This equals approximately 131 million people, and the number continues to climb. Thirty-five percent of patients diagnosed as overweight are 35 years of age or younger. Most have tried diets at one time or another, and 95 percent are unsuccessful at losing weight and keeping it off, even for a short time. Your odds of permanent weight loss on a "diet" are only a little better than your chance of becoming an astronaut. What does this mean to you? Are you destined to be overweight all your life? Absolutely not! You need only learn the principles of a healthy lifestyle and live by those basic principles.

Health and weight management are the first things to get set aside and become neglected in one's life. Do you remember the times that you started an exercise program and then became "too busy" to stick with the plan? We are all guilty of short-term false starts. The speed of life makes many priorities go by the wayside. But fitness and health must be the foundation of your life. Those who make health the foundation of their lives create rich, splendid lives. Imagine neglecting your career; how well would that go? How long would you keep your job if you didn't do much work or didn't even show up? Wouldn't you be fired before long? What about your family?

If you neglected them, wouldn't your relationships suffer turmoil — if they continued to exist at all?

If you lose your health, the rest of your life will be set aside, and your focus will become survival. That is especially true as we age. Without a healthy, strong body, senior citizens exhaust nearly all their energy simply surviving. Often people who neglect their health spend their final years bedridden or incapacitated. The closing acts of so many people's lives are wasted because they lived in the moment without ever considering the future. That is no way to end your time on Earth. Instead of spending all of your energy just surviving, you can thrive at any age. Leonardo da Vinci, Thomas Edison, Charles Darwin, and many other masterminds asserted that a strong and healthy body is mandatory for a full and complete life. Without health, nothing else matters.

A BETTER WAY

We all want different things. Whether your goal is to maintain a fit lifestyle or to lose weight and create the body of a fitness model, you can achieve it. You might be fighting the battle of the bulge (and gravity), or you might be severely overweight and don't know what to do about it. You might be ready to give up after many failed attempts at losing weight. So many people feel as if they have tried everything. The airwaves are flooded with claims that you can have a model's body without getting off the couch. BULL! Don't fall prey to these ridiculous claims!

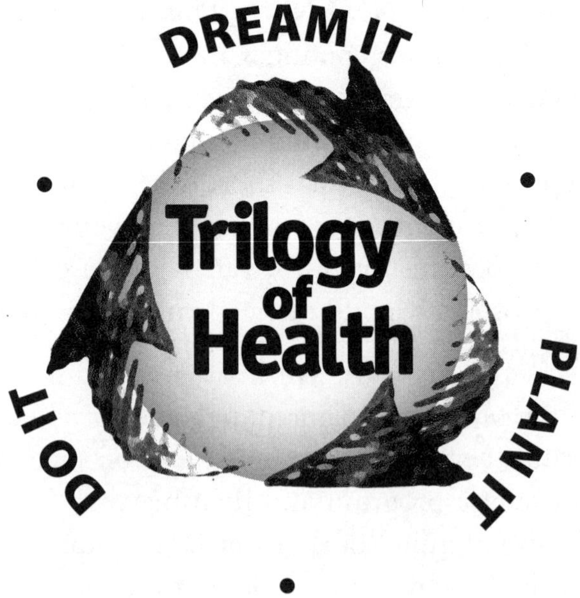

DREAM IT, PLAN IT, DO IT

Everything starts with a dream. To make a dream reality you must make it the foundation of your life and create a plan. When the plan is put into action your dreams become a reality.

You will learn to achieve a fundamental physical and emotional change. The *BetterBody*

BetterLife program is an all-natural lifestyle management plan designed to take less than 3 percent of your day. It is based on the philosophy of the *Trilogy of Health*. When a person commits to the three fundamentals of healthy living — proper nutrition, cardiovascular conditioning, and muscle toning — he or she maximizes the ability to live a long, fit, and healthy life.

And yes, this can all be done in less than 3 percent of your day.

FOUNDATION OF YOUR LIFE

Create a strong body and mind; then build your life on top of that foundation. A concrete foundation is not strong enough to support a house unless the mixture was formulated from all three of its components: cement, sand, and water. If the builder leaves out one of the elements, the foundation will crumble. In the same way, the human body will fall into disrepair without a *Trilogy of Health* foundation: nutrition, cardiovascular conditioning, and muscle toning must all be present and in proper balance for the body to be effective and strong. A healthy and fit body is requisite to a sound mind, soul, and life. The body is the foundation for all activities. Create the best foundation for life and reap limitless rewards.

When I was a child, my friends and I used to ride our bicycles to Joe's Corner Store. We called it the candy store because we went there for candy. Joe looked after us, and we patronized his store with great regularity. Times were simpler then. Across the street from the candy store stood an old Federalist Victorian house, the mansion of the neighborhood at four thousand square feet. My friends and I would sit on the bench in front of Joe's and talk about the big house. Four massive columns reached toward the sky and supported the front-porch roof. With its majestic mahogany veranda and wrought-iron railings, the home towered over the sloping front yard and once-earthen roads. We imagined a family of great importance standing on the balcony and waving good morning to those walking by. It was an impressive structure to be sure. As the years passed, however, the house began to show signs of wear, but they were ignored. The house continued to fall apart until it was an abandoned shell of what it once was.

Your body is like that house. If you neglect your home, it will rot and decay. So will your body. Years go by and we get older. The neglected body begins to break down, but we ignore the signs and the situation grows worse. Soon the weight piles on, fitness declines, and health deteriorates.

Soon a single flight of stairs makes you out of breath, and a heart attack is only one fast-food burger or stressful day away. Much like the house across from the candy store, years of apathy turn your body into a shell of what it once was.

It's never too late to start. You can begin a better way of living that will help you get the body and life that you deserve, using a natural program built on the fundamentals of human physiology. You can easily adapt what you will learn from this book to your lifestyle, your schedule, and your life. You will change your life forever.

THE RIGHT PATH

On life's journey, you have many choices, and you can follow many different paths. You can take the path of the masses — eating unhealthy fast food, having a sedentary lifestyle, and complaining about being overweight — or you can take the path of an active and healthy life. Living healthily and naturally is a great path, presenting a wonderful view and many great opportunities. It will also make life's journey pleasurable and long. You will accomplish more than you have ever dreamed on your day-by-day travels. Your life will be so much more enjoyable and full. You will thank me, and your loved ones will thank you.

"Live life to the fullest. You have only one chance and only one body. Don't waste either of them."

SUMMARY

- Diets do not work. They are temporary and ineffective.
- Healthy and fit living requires less than 3 percent of your day.
- The *Trilogy of Health* will make achieving and enjoying a healthy body easy, possible, and permanent.
- The *BetterBody BetterLife* program is simple and natural. It is based on the fundamentals of human physiology.
- A fit and healthy body is prerequisite to a sound mind, soul, and life.

Chapter Two

INCREASE YOUR ODDS

We are judged by our appearance. We are evaluated by how we dress, groom our hair, speak, gesture, and look. Unfortunately, that is how our world functions, how workplaces operate, and how relationships start — or don't start. Our appearance determines whether we are taken seriously or taken advantage of. Every day we are judged before we can utter a single word.

JUDGING BY APPEARANCES

When you walk into an auto dealership, every salesperson judges the odds of your buying a car. Salespeople "size up" your potential; they assess your car, clothes, and behavior. After observing for a few moments, the salesperson will decide either to offer you assistance or to hide in the coffee room. When that salesperson walks in your direction, you do the same thing. Does this person appear qualified? Is he or she dressed appropriately? Are mannerisms consistent with honest salespersons you've met in the past?

During a job interview, the same two-way critiquing takes place. The interviewer judges more than an applicant's résumé. Appearance, attire, and attitude are important, too. Often a candidate with fewer qualifications is hired based on nothing more than appearance. Physical appearance is particularly critical in promotion to upper-management and high-profile positions. It is a reflection of an employee's credibility as a balanced person in business and personal life. An overweight employee has external signs of a life out of balance. Employers consider physical appearance an indicator of a worker's value. They may not be wrong in doing so. Several studies have documented that overweight people use more sick days and have more issues that interfere with job performance than do employees of a healthy weight. The scrutiny does not end off the job. At social gatherings, people often decide to talk to you, or not, because of the way you look. As much as we would like to believe that this doesn't happen, it does.

You might be wondering why I am painting such a picture of gloom. I don't mean to sound bleak. The world is an incredible and intriguing place, in part due to appearances. Our differences bring color and variety to life. Nonetheless, those who are overweight are often seen for their size before they are seen as a person. This prejudice is as strong as any other. A few people are happy to be large, and their size fits into their lifestyles. Since you are reading this program, I know you are not one of those people; you want to change your body. You have realized that excess weight is stopping you from getting everything out of life that you can. You have limited not only your mobility and your energy, but also your life span. Odds are that your family feels the same way; nobody wants a parent, child, sibling, or spouse to be overweight and unhealthy.

New Worlds

With this plan, you can have a healthier body and a great physique. You can have abundant energy, and new worlds will open up to you. When you get into good physical shape, you will want to do more things — probably things that you never desired before. You won't be embarrassed by the way you look in an outfit or in a bathing suit. When people lose weight and get into good physical condition, they often find themselves wanting to attain even better shape and to progress even further.

As reported in *Runner's World* online, Elijah Lagat was told by his doctor a little over a decade ago that he was 35 pounds overweight and in poor physical condition. He was told that fat deposits were forming on his heart and that he should exercise because his current condition was putting his life in jeopardy of a heart attack. He started jogging with the intention of simply losing some weight. He was so embarrassed in the beginning that he jogged at night so nobody would see him. A few years later, he ran in some local races, and he even won a few. He then went on to enter more competitive races, and in 1997, he won the Berlin Marathon. He didn't plan to run marathons in the beginning; he only needed to drop the excess weight. Elijah Lagat went on to win the 2000 Boston Marathon.

The great success story of Sam Gadless was reported on Sportsillustrated.CNN.com. Sam was unhealthy all his life. He was a chain smoker with high cholesterol; he had borderline adult onset diabetes and severe arthritis. When his doctor told him that his days were numbered, he started reading and learning. He became active in resurrecting his body when in his seventies. In 1992, at age 85, Sam ran and completed his first New York City Marathon. In 1995, his son and grandson joined him, and they now run as a family, Team Gadless. Sam went on to complete his seventh NYC Marathon at age 91. Families that exercise together stay fit together.

Will you be the next amazing success story? Life is too short not to take good care of your body. Life is too short not to enjoy it to the fullest. It is never too late to take back your life with a healthy body, healthy mind, and healthy soul.

"You have only one body, and there are no trade-ins! Isn't it time to start your restoration?"

SUMMARY

- We're judged by our appearances and mannerisms.
- Those who are overweight are often seen for their size before they are seen as individuals.
- You can have a great physique and a healthier body, and break past the the barrier of being overwieght .
- You can take back your life and become the next success story.

Chapter Three

IN THE COMPANY OF OTHERS

Your family and friends love you and they want the best for you. When you tell them about an idea or project, they may oppose it: "That will never work. I tried that" or "I know this woman at work who did that and she hated it." It is not that your friends or family want you to fail. Often they are trying to protect you from failure and do not want to see you get hurt. Because most people fail at losing weight and keeping it off on a diet, others assume you will fail too. The odds are against you with a diet. Good thing the *BetterBody BetterLife* plan is not a diet.

Misery loves company. People will often hit you when you are down. They may not mean to, or they may be doing it at a subconscious level, but it happens. One of my favorite philosophies comes from a Tony Robbins seminar. Tony explains that there are two ways to own the tallest building in town. Either you can tear down all of the taller buildings, or you can build the tallest one. Some people tear down others to feel better about themselves. You are better than that, so you need to focus on building your building taller and staying away from those who choose to tear others down. Some close friends or relatives may not want you to succeed because subconsciously they are afraid that they will not have the same relationship with you when you achieve your goal. That can be especially true if you are in a family or circle of friends in which everyone is overweight.

When I tell some people about an idea, many respond with sarcasm and tell me that my idea won't work. They react negatively because they are averse to change or risk. It is easier to say that something won't work than it is to get off your duff to see if it will. Pessimism can be equated to laziness. I now surround myself with "possibility people."

We expect friends and family members to support the things that we want to do. If someone close to you is not supportive of your plan to change your life, do not discuss your plans; talk about other things. I am not saying that you should keep secrets, only that you should pick your battles wisely and your topics of discussion with prudence. Choose as sounding boards those people who are supportive and truthful. Choose people who will help you build a taller building.

Do You Have a Fan Club?

When you start to lose weight and look better, everyone will have a new outlook about you and what you have done. As you lose weight, friends, family members, and coworkers will want to know what diet you are on. When you tell them that you are not "on a diet," they may express disbelief. Americans have the misconception that you have to diet, or starve yourself, to lose weight and be thin. Don't be bashful about explaining how you are doing it. Be boastful that you are simply living a better lifestyle and taking better care of yourself. Be your own biggest fan.

Sports teams prefer to play in their hometown because they have the home-team advantage. The familiarity of the field, the short journey to the game, the crowd that cheers for them, and the love of friends and family all promote better performance. Sports teams have fans. You need fans, too. Avoid those who say, "That will never work." Seek out those who support you, believe in you, and want to see you succeed. Surround yourself with these people and make them your fan club!

When you talk with a nonfan who asks, "How's it going?" answer, "Fantastic, and it's getting better." Do not engage in detailed conversation with a skeptic. In time that person may see that you are succeeding and achieving your dreams, and he or she may become part of your support team, your fan club. Until then, keep your distance. You need — we all need — to be around people who truly care for us and want us to realize our dreams. Don't make your journey any harder than it has to be. Find those who will push, motivate, and encourage you to reach your goals.

Meet with your fan club or speak with its members often. Have a "fan club night" once a month with your biggest fans. Let them know how you are doing; relate your successes and areas for imporvement. Share in their successes, too. Your fans will boost you higher and help pick you up when you need a hand. You can return the favor. You can be there for others when they need you. Pick them up when they are down, raise them higher when they are successful, and love them when they need a shoulder to rest on. When you are giving to someone, you are also receiving.

Ah, but what if you do not have any fans? At times, everyone is short of fans. You may have moved, changed jobs, or modified your life. View such changes as a great opportunity to build a new fan club. If you are building a fit body, join a fitness club and talk with others; you will probably find several people that you click with. Invite your fans over for coffee and tell them to bring their fans. Go online into forums or chat rooms. A fan does not have to be someone you meet face to face. The newest idea that I love is using www.youtube.com to find fans. People are now creating videoblogs, connecting with others of like mind and meeting new best friends. You can also check local community message boards for events with people of like mind. You can locate social groups in your area on Internet sites such as www.meetup.com. If you want something to happen, you must go out and make it happen. Build your home-team advantage by building a rich and diverse fan club!

THE GREATEST SATISFACTION

Your journey will be your greatest satisfaction. The old dilapidated house across from Joe's candy store eventually went into foreclosure after many years of neglect and abuse. Even at the foreclosure auction, many building contractors passed on the opportunity to purchase the house because of its condition. I called the bank the next day and submitted an offer that they accepted. I became the proud owner of the money pit.

When I started the rehabilitation project, I had a vision of what the house would look like when I was done, just as you should have a vision of what you will look like when you have accomplished your weight-loss and fitness goals. I enthusiastically showed the house to all my friends and family before I started. Everyone laughed at me; my family thought I was crazy, and my friends said there was no way I could do it. The house had been severely damaged by a fire. The second floor was gutted, and all the windows had been missing for years. Necessities were absent, including a kitchen, working plumbing, and electricity.

What's more, the basement had 2 feet of water standing in it, and the attic was home to pigeons and hundreds of bats. The house was uninhabitable. Most people said it should have been torn down.

I worked on the house from 4 to 6 hours every night (after working all day), and I worked every weekend for 12 to 15 hours a day. The resurrection slowly began; I wouldn't let anyone hold me back. The renovation of that house was the most severe financial strain and the hardest emotional battle of my life, but the vision that I had from the beginning led me to the finish; it kept me going through the worst of times, and it provided the highest of glories. The satisfaction of success was priceless.

Often, after years of neglect, we find our bodies ready to go into foreclosure. Don't let that happen. You, too, have to hold a vision in your mind of what you want, and you have to work toward that vision every day. See in your mind how you will look and feel, but remember that results do not happen overnight. Work to achieve your goals and earn the satisfaction of success with your body. There is no feeling in this world that can compare to what you will feel when you look in the mirror and see the temple that you have worked to build and the healthy body that is the foundation of your life. Every morning you will look in the mirror as you get dressed, and you will be thrilled because you will be reminded of your effort and dedication. There will be no need to fret over which outfit makes you look fat; none will. You will say, "I did it!" And then you will agree with me that there is no greater satisfaction than achieving your goals.

"Whether you think you can or you think you can't, you're right."

AUTHOR UNKNOWN

SUMMARY

- Surround yourself with people who will support your goals and plans.
- Create your own fan club.
- The only person who can stop you from achieving whatever you desire is you.
- Have a vision and work toward it every day.

Chapter Four

IT'S ALL ABOUT ATTITUDE

Do people have a great attitude because they are doing well, or are they doing well because they have a great attitude? Attitude comes first! Life is attitude and your perception of the world. A positive attitude is a common denominator among high achievers; they are optimistic and genuinely happy no matter what the situation.

A POSITIVE ATTITUDE IS A CHOICE!

Do you have a problem? I don't believe in problems, only challenges and obstacles. When a negative situation arises, most people say that they have a problem. The only problem is the belief that the "situation" is a problem. Problems are simply challenges to conquer or obstacles to remove from your life. You are reading this program because you have a challenge to overcome. You will get past one of the toughest challenges in your life while having fun. When you eradicate the weight and health obstacle, you will see many other obstacles disappearing simultaneously. Your life will become fuller and more enjoyable, and your horizons will expand.

LUCK FAVORS THE WELL PREPARED

How many times have you heard, "With my [bad] luck..."? I want you to eliminate that statement from your speech. It is one of the worst phrases that can be spoken. Everyone has luck, mostly good but some bad. "Luck favors the well prepared." I believe that, and I live by it. For example, if you take driving lessons to learn the proper techniques, drive carefully, and own a safe, well-engineered car, then you reduce your chances of having an auto accident. However, if you are an inexperienced driver who has never taken a lesson and you drive a poorly maintained car, you are much more likely to get into an accident. Luck is directly proportionate to the level of preparedness. The more you are prepared, the better luck you will have. When I bought the old, dilapidated home I affectionately called the money pit, I drew architectural plans and schematics. I knew I would make more mistakes and take longer to finish the project if I wasn't prepared with good plans.

Don't think of an unfortunate occurrence as bad luck. Consider it good luck that things aren't worse. There is always an unseen benefit; you only have to look for it. Many people have good luck but view it as bad luck. For example, an auto accident might be viewed as bad luck. Yes, it was an unfortunate event, but a winner would see surviving it as good luck. The outcome could have been far worse. Every day that you wake up to experience the miracle of being alive you have good luck — incredible, miraculous luck. Every day you wake up is an amazing day and a new start. Unfortunate events are just that, unfortunate events. Unfortunate events are also "positive negative feedback." In other words, "bad luck" can teach you how to do something differently or how to be better prepared next time. Be thankful for every gift, even the tiniest ones. Don't miss the silver lining in the cloud, even if you have to chase after it.

For example, if you find yourself eating garbage food or skipping exercise, don't beat yourself up over it. Be happy that you understand and recognize that you are off your path to health. You are lucky to have that conscious thought and to be able to act on it — not "later" or "tomorrow," but in the moment. You must act on it NOW to change the pattern.

Here's an example. You realize that you are finishing your third cupcake. You are eating it because a pattern has been etched in your brain for years. If you change the pattern the moment it occurs, you make substantial progress toward permanently changing it. Stop eating. Get the rest of the box and the half-eaten cupcake in your hand. Throw them on the ground and jump up and down on them. Crush them into a disgusting mess and then throw them into the garbage. From then on, every time you consider eating a cupcake, you will see in your mind the crushed cupcakes and you will remember the pain that they caused you. Now you are lucky! An acronym for L.U.C.K. is Labor Under Constructive Knowledge.

So how do you become well prepared? Learn everything you can to make living a healthy lifestyle easy. Use common sense and be cautious. In order to keep selling magazines or products, many publishers, equipment manufacturers, and supplement companies use new twists to gain a competitive edge. Diet and exercise fads are a way to stand out from the crowd. I am not saying that it's wrong...uh, yes I am. Fancy new exercise products are unnecessarily complicated for most beginners — and even for experts. Many diet products are simply bad advice, coming from entrepreneurs out to make a buck without concern for your health. Even the government's food pyramid is tainted and biased because the food industry and its lobbyists are protecting their profits.

A healthy lifestyle is simple, logical, and effective. I have based my program on the fundamentals of human physiology. I have designed it to be simple and straightforward because easy steps will help you follow through. Simple equals success.

Time Management

Part of being well prepared is time management. If you do not plan an adequate amount of time to complete tasks, you are destined to fail before you start. The speed of life will push your dreams by the wayside. Schedule your fitness time as you would any other event or meeting. Scheduling will almost guarantee that you don't miss it. Keep exercise on the top of the list by completing it before the rest of your day starts. If I don't exercise in the morning, I usually miss it that day. My lapse is not intentional, but I generally do not have enough time or motivation at the end of the day. So called "emergencies" arise frequently; they can throw your schedule into disarray. The morning is also the most effective time of day to exercise. Morning exercise gives the body a natural boost. Morning exercise helps you feel more alert, deal with stress more efficiently, and have more energy throughout the day. A few minutes of exercise in the morning will keep you feeling great for the 16 hours that follow. There are few better investments.

Start a ritual that will get you raring to go every single day. When you wake up, sit up at the end of your bed, and take three slow and deep breaths. Breathing is the essence of life. Then say out loud in a convincing voice (because your mind and the language you use will shape your life),

"Today is going to be an incredible day because I can make it that way!

I will lead my day with balance and healthy living.

I will believe and achieve.

I have control of my choices and I will choose well.

I am the leader of my life.

I control my destiny."

Then go exercise immediately. After you exercise, eat a balanced and nutritious breakfast. After starting this routine, you will find that you have energy to go all day and still have enough energy for your children and your hobbies. You may even go out to dinner with friends and not fall asleep at the table. At first this routine requires effort to adjust your schedule, but your rewards will be better sleep, increased productivity, and greater energy.

Energy Boost

A few weeks into the *BetterBody BetterLife* program, you will feel better. Your energy level will increase dramatically. With your energy rising and your body transforming, your attitude will shine. When those around you start to notice that you have lost weight and have more energy, they will ask what your secret is. You will get excited and your attitude will radiate. When you can live your life with more energy than ever before, your outlook will improve even more. This will be contagious. The people in your life will start to catch your better attitude; in return, you will enjoy better relationships. Attitude is contagious.

Life is about mind-set and perspective on the world. If your perspective is sour, then your life will be sour. If your mind-set is grand, then your life will be filled with excitement and pleasure. That is why someone with little can be happy, and someone with many riches can be miserable. The old saying that money can't buy you happiness is true. Your attitude, perspective, and approach toward life determine your happiness, with or without money.

"The only problem in life is viewing events as problems. Life does not have problems, only challenges, which can be overcome."

SUMMARY

- Attitude is first and foremost. It determines your response to every event in life.
- There are no problems, only challenges and obstacles.
- View events as good luck. Find the silver lining.
- Be well prepared. Knowledge and time management are key.
- Life is about mind-set. Let yours be grand.
- A positive attitude is a choice!

Chapter Five

AVOID THE RISKS

Complications from obesity kill over 6,000 people in the U.S. every day.

Do you want to die 20 years before your time? It is well known that being overweight leads to an increased level of health risks. Those risks might be one reason that you are reading this program. The diseases and risks that are linked to being overweight are numerous and horrible. They are among the reasons that I turned to a healthy lifestyle. I have a high risk of cardiac complications and adult onset diabetes because of my heredity, and I don't care to experience the series of events that I have seen my relatives endure. I have vowed to do all that is possible not to suffer those horrific diseases. If you are hostage to similar bloodlines, you too can greatly increase your chances of overcoming your hereditary risks.

Studies involving millions of people have shown that mortality is lowest in healthy, nonsmoking men 20 to 69 years of age who are less than 5 percent overweight; and among women ages 30 to 69 who are less than 15 percent overweight. One long-term study concluded that, for every pound of excess weight, the risk of mortality increases by 1 percent for those younger than 50. At age 50, the death rate increases by 2 percent for each extra pound.

In addition, most studies show an increase in mortality rate associated with obesity. Obesity is clinically defined as being more than 20 percent overweight, or having a BMI (Body Mass Index, see page 216) of 30 or more. Obese individuals have a 50 to 100 percent increased risk of death from all causes compared with healthy-weight individuals (BMI of 20-25). Most of the increased risk arises from cardiovascular causes.

The greater the excess weight, the shorter the life expectancy.

MEDICAL ISSUES THAT CAN ARISE FROM PHYSICAL AND DIETARY NEGLECT:

Cancer (certain forms)

Women
- Breast
- Uterine
- Ovarian
- Gallbladder

Men
- Colon
- Rectal
- Prostate

Cardiovascular diseases
- High blood pressure
- Arteriosclerosis
- Atherosclerosis
- High cholesterol

Respiratory Disorders
- Respiratory difficulties
- Pickwickian Syndrome
- Sleep apnea

Diabetes (type II adult onset)

Musculoskeletal Problems
- Arthritis
- Osteoarthritis
- Back problems
- Degenerative disc diseases
- Joint dysfunctions
- Foot problems
- Mobility limitations

Other Possible Complications
- Depression
- Social stigma
- Social anxiety
- Activity limitations
- Chemical dependency
- Sexual dysfunction

Avoid the Risks

This is a somber and dreadful subject, but the facts are well known throughout the medical community. If you are overweight — and certainly if you are obese — your risks of disease are substantially higher than those of your fit counterpart. Being overweight and obese WILL cause medical problems.

Unhealthy living habits, combined with heredity, can put you in a high-risk category. In many cases, losing weight reduces, relieves, or eliminates poor health. That alone should be enough to persuade anyone to lose weight and live a healthier life.

I do not know anyone who has said, "I want to be really fat, have adult onset diabetes, get clogged arteries, and go through three cardiac surgeries to try to fix them, but then die before my child graduates from high school." Do you?

It is not my goal to frighten you, but if I have...well, good. You should be scared. These are the facts, and the best way to avoid these horrors is to eat right and stay active.

Excess body fat accelerates the aging process. Think about this: How many elderly people who are overweight look their age? Don't they look older? How many can participate in physical activities or simply move without difficulty? I am drawing your attention to the fact that most elderly people could still be dancing, playing tennis, or doing anything else that they might choose. You can be active into your nineties and beyond. Do you want to spend your fifties, sixties, and seventies using most of your energy just moving? Simply getting up out of a chair is difficult for many. Most people grow old before their time — WAY before their time.

As a volunteer emergency medical technician, I have seen many people who would not need my assistance if they were of a healthy weight. Most would not have the medical complications they have if they lived a healthy lifestyle. You can live a long, healthy, and active life, or you can grow old and obese and regret your choices until your last day. The decision is yours.

Taking care of your body is like taking care of an old house. The first signs of wear and deterioration are unseen and undetected, but the decay is occurring. A house shows decay with rotten wood and a leaky roof; the failing body deteriorates with high blood pressure, excess weight, and high cholesterol. A quick fix for both is attempted, but the caulk on the roof and the fad diets fail in a short time. The house sags and crumbles from rot and corrosion. The body weakens with diabetes or heart attacks. Soon the house is torn down, and the body is put into the ground.

It is not too late to take control of your health and rebuild the house that you live in 24 hours a day and 7 days a week.

"Obesity is the second leading cause of preventable death in America."

DR. C. EVERETT KOOP, FORMER SURGEON GENERAL OF THE UNITED STATES

SUMMARY

- Being overweight or obese causes medical problems.
- Each pound of excess weight increases the risk of death.
- Heredity can increase medical risks. When combined with excess body fat, risks become a certainty.
- By achieving and maintaining a healthier body and lifestyle, you can be active longer and enjoy a better quality of life.

Chapter Six

NATURE VS. NURTURE

Few events in your life are beyond your control. Nearly everything that happens to adults results from their actions, reactions, or inactions. You can influence, if not control, virtually every affair in your life. Think about your life. Is there anything that you cannot control? For example, you can avoid speeding tickets by obeying the speed limit. You can improve your grades in school by studying more. You can achieve a fit body with a healthful lifestyle. You cannot control others, and you cannot control some events, but you can control your choices.

Don't beat yourself up because of your choices, but learn from them and recognize that you can change anything in your life that you desire. Good or bad, your life is the way it is because you created it or allowed it to happen. And those few things that are beyond our control, we can choose the meaning that we attach to them. Nothing has meaning until we give it meaning. We all need to take responsibility for the events in our lives. If you don't, you will not get the things you want, you will never be the person you want to be, and you will never have the happiness that you crave. Taking responsibility is how we improve ourselves and evolve into better people. Generally, people do not take the time to analyze their actions or reactions, and therefore they rarely improve. Socrates said it best: "The unexamined life is not worth living."

NATURE

Nature has given most of us one health risk or another. We are born that way; it is in our genes. We also have the circumstances of our lives that trigger health problems. This is commonly referred to as "nature vs. nurture." Nature gives us the things that we cannot control. Our DNA, the genes that we received from our parents, controls our physical characteristics (for example, height, hair color, bone structure, blood type, and more). Incredibly, some inborn risk factors can be minimized or eliminated with exercise and balanced dietary practices.

NURTURE

Nurture refers to environmental factors in our lives and includes nearly everything we experience. Where we live and work, what we eat, how we speak, the way we were raised, the friends we choose, and our dietary behaviors are just a few. These factors often dictate our habits. Habits are formed early in life and they continue throughout maturity. Most of the things that we do are habits, conditioned behaviors that we learned by watching and learning from the actions of others. Other habits are formed because we are filling a human need. Habits are not limited to eating. Most of our actions are learned and conditioned responses. The old adage "The apple does not fall far from the tree," has some validity. If a parent is active in a hobby, a child will often have the same hobby in adult life. Children often follow their parent's example. Children of doctors often become doctors; children of mechanics often become mechanics; and children of overweight parents tend to be overweight. We learn and act in a similar fashion to the people who are close to us. If you hang out with fat people who don't care about health or fitness, then you are likely to remain overweight, too. On the other hand, if you hang out with people who are committed to losing weight and getting healthy, then you, too, are likely to lose weight and become healthy. There is a saying, "You are the average of the people you are around the most." Who are you hanging out with?

GROWING PAINS

Most of us have preconceived notions about how we should live our lives, when we should marry, which career we should choose, and much more. Unless you grew up in a health-conscious family, you probably didn't give fitness much thought after high school physical education classes. An unfortunate deficit in our school system is the lack of health and fitness education. We were all required to attend physical education (gym) classes, but we were not taught about being fit. We played dodge ball instead. Most of us did not receive a meaningful education in how to live healthily. The result is that two-thirds of Americans are overweight.

You know that you should be active and eat well, but you never learned what that really means. Surely, you have an idea. Almost every day you hear news about the latest diets or exercises, which are usually fads, but you are not sure how to be fit and healthy. I will be the last one to say that it is not your fault that you are overweight, because nobody is forcing you to sit around all day and eat garbage food. However, the blame for our epidemic of obesity also rests on the shoulders of government, the schools, and parents because they are the gatekeepers of information. You can break this cycle! You can make a difference in your life, your family, your children, and your friends. You can be the catalyst of change.

Most families do not instill in their children the importance of eating right. That failure, in part, can be attributed to the parents' lack of health and fitness knowledge. How often is a child's first solid food a McDonald's French fry or part of a greasy cheeseburger? Younger generations are growing up on fast food and eating on the run. Double-income families often opt for takeout and microwave meals due to time restrictions. As a result, many young adults don't cook; some never learn. They end up living on supersized fast food, nuked meals, cereal, and takeout. There is not much of a chance of having a healthy diet if you do that.

Older generations grew up learning not to waste — to eat everything on their plates. They, in turn, gave their children large portions and encouraged them to have seconds. Does this sound familiar? How do you eat now? Many people don't believe that they have had enough to eat until they get that bloated feeling. Many of us were taught to accept seconds so we wouldn't offend the chef. Do you do this when you are at your in-laws' or a friend's house? These habits have been nurtured since we were toddlers.

KNOWLEDGE EQUALS POTENTIAL CHANGE

Unless we make a conscious effort to educate ourselves and then implement that knowledge, we will not get different results. The definition of insanity is doing the same things over and over but expecting different results. You will not get a different result if you do not do different things.

You must never stop learning, never stop improving, and never give less than a valiant effort. Since I graduated from college, I have spent more money on education than I spent in a typical year of college. Every year I take several specialized 2- to 6-day intensive training courses to increase my knowledge and experience. I also have coaches in many different areas of expertise. These people keep me on track and push me through my comfort zone to get to the next level; they assure that I follow through. I am dedicated to lifelong learning because I believe if you're not growing, you're dying.

Knowledge and information are worthless without action. The way to achieve change is through education, persistence, and action. You may be thinking, "Easy for you to say, Croix, you have the time and money to get great training and coaching." We all have the same 24 hours in a day; it is a matter of how we prioritize those 24 hours. I understand the importance of constantly improving, so I make time in my schedule. Education has always been a financial stretch for me. I paid my way through college working full time, and I continue to stretch my budget to increase my education. Every time I do, I grow as a person and grow in my career.

Some of the ways to increase your knowledge and experience are free or very inexpensive. Reading books is free if you go to the library; books can be purchased at low cost also. One of the greatest and free ways to improve your life is to analyze the efforts and actions of each day and learn from them. Learn from your mistakes so they don't happen again. Repeat your successes. You can change any aspect of your life. Observe others and learn from them, too. You can overcome anything that you were conditioned to do as a child or adult and replace the bad habits with good ones. What choices have you made that have positively affected your life? What choices have you made that have negatively affected your life? Your choices matter, so choose carefully.

SUCCESS IS IN YOUR FUTURE. CAN YOU SEE IT?

"The unexamined life is not worth living."

SOCRATES

SUMMARY

- You can control virtually every event in your life.
- Nature is the aspects of ourselves that we cannot change (for example, hair color, height, blood type).
- Nurture is everything that we experience and do — the events we CAN change.
- Nearly everything that we do is a conditioned habit or response.
- You can change any aspect of your life by analyzing actions and reactions and by making a constant effort to improve.
- Change is achieved through education, persistence, and action.

Chapter Seven

GETTING STARTED

Where to start? Many people find this the hardest part. Some people don't have a clear idea of what they want; others don't know how to take that first step. As you read on, you will learn effective methods for figuring out what you want, getting started, and staying on track. Your first step will often determine the level of your success. Follow these steps and you can succeed. Each step is important and necessary. Success will come from using each step and building upon the steps to create the whole plan. Success is not achieved by accident; success is achieved by design.

KEEPING RECORDS

You will need a notebook or a journal, one that you will keep permanently. This is part of your foundation because you need the ability to refer back to what you've done, motivate yourself, and monitor your progress. You need to track what you are doing. Your record can be as simple as short, handwritten notes on a note pad.

Many studies have shown that those who have written qualitative and quantitative goals are more successful than those who don't. They attain their goals with greater frequency and precision. Those who keep a record of their journey toward their goals are significantly more likely to succeed, and they are more able to adapt or change to assure consistent progress.

This trend is especially true in weight loss and fitness management. The majority of those who are successful in permanent weight loss are the ones who keep a journal of exercise and dietary consumption. It is often the difference between a true desire to succeed and merely wishing.

You can use an ordinary notebook, your computer, or the *BetterBody BetterLife Journal* that I have designed for this program. It will get you started and take you through the first 3 months of your journey. It is formatted to motivate you through the steps and to help ensure your success. Keep your notebook or journal with you as you go through the program. Your journal will contain your master list of goals, your plan to achieve your goals, and a record of your progress. The possibilities are limited only by your imagination and commitment.

BETTERBODY BETTERLIFE JOURNAL

The first step toward your success is to know what you want. Does that statement sound funny to you? It seems obvious and elementary. Many people think that they know what they want, but in reality, they have only a vague idea, or they have nothing more than wishes and dreams. If you have not thoroughly considered all your dreams and wishes, written them down, prioritized them, set goals based on them, and made a plan to achieve them, then your desires are still just dreams and wishes. If a wish stays a wish or a dream stays a dream, it will never be realized. "I wish I could lose weight," or "I wish that I had a body like hers." On the other hand, when you write down your wish or your dream, you are taking the first step toward turning that wish into a goal. Goals can then be turned into a plan, and plans can be achieved with action and persistence. Whoa, we are getting ahead of ourselves! There is a little more to making your dreams happen than just writing down your dreams, but one step at a time. Remember, everything starts with a dream, and anything is possible with a vision and a plan.

Open the *BetterBody BetterLife Journal to "Dreams to Goals:* ***Worksheet****"* on page 53. Write down what you want — your dreams and your wishes. (Page 54 will stay blank for now.) We will limit this exercise to fitness and health issues, but make no mistake, this goal-setting and planning process will work for all aspects of your life. If you know what you want, then write your goals at the top of the second page in the journal. If you are not sure, write down any fitness wishes that come to mind and ponder your list until you have several ideas for goals.

I asked my friend Amy to allow us to follow her as she learns how to set goals and live a healthy life. Amy is a 35-year-old mother with a wonderful 4-year-old daughter. She works full time as an elementary school teacher in a busy suburban New England town. Her husband works for the town where they live. Amy has always been a few pounds over her ideal weight, and as she approached her late twenties, her weight slowly increased. Amy also gained some weight during her pregnancy and didn't lose it all after the baby arrived. Now at age 35, she weighs 30 pounds more than she did when she graduated from college. Amy's dietary habits have been fair throughout her life; however, she has been prone to snacking, and she has a weak spot for chocolate desserts. Amy's example shows only six of her goals, but you may have more. Write down every one of them.

GOALS TO DREAMS
WORKSHEET

Eat better

Lose 30 pounds

Live healthy

Learn to dance

Learn to swim

Exercise more

Your goals might be to lose weight and get into good physical condition. Maybe you wrote down "learn how to dance." You may not have learned to dance because of your weight. This is a great goal to write. Now look at the whole list and study it carefully. Does the list seem to show the ideals in your life? If it doesn't, go back and spend a little more time on this part. It is very important and cannot be skipped. You should list every health and fitness goal that you want to achieve in the future, in both the short- and long-term. If you have not made your list yet, start now.

If you need to add to or change your list, you can do so at any time. You could even have an ambitious desire to complete a 5-kilometer run or even a triathlon. Did you notice that I said complete? I didn't say win. I said this because many people enter to finish, not to beat anyone else. My goals for my first few triathlons were to finish without injuries and not come in last. I came in number 141 out of 143 in one of my early attempts. The idea that you can complete and finish is exhilarating enough; it helps you to stay focused when getting ready for the events. I always get an emotional and physical high after a triathlon. Finishing is winning!

Look at what you wrote and decide which goals are most important to you. Prioritize and number them in order. Next, rewrite your list in the prioritized order below your first list. This will be your goal list. When you rewrite your goals, always write in the positive. Your goals should be written as "I will" statements and be quantified if possible: for example, "I will lose 30 pounds." You now have a goal list.

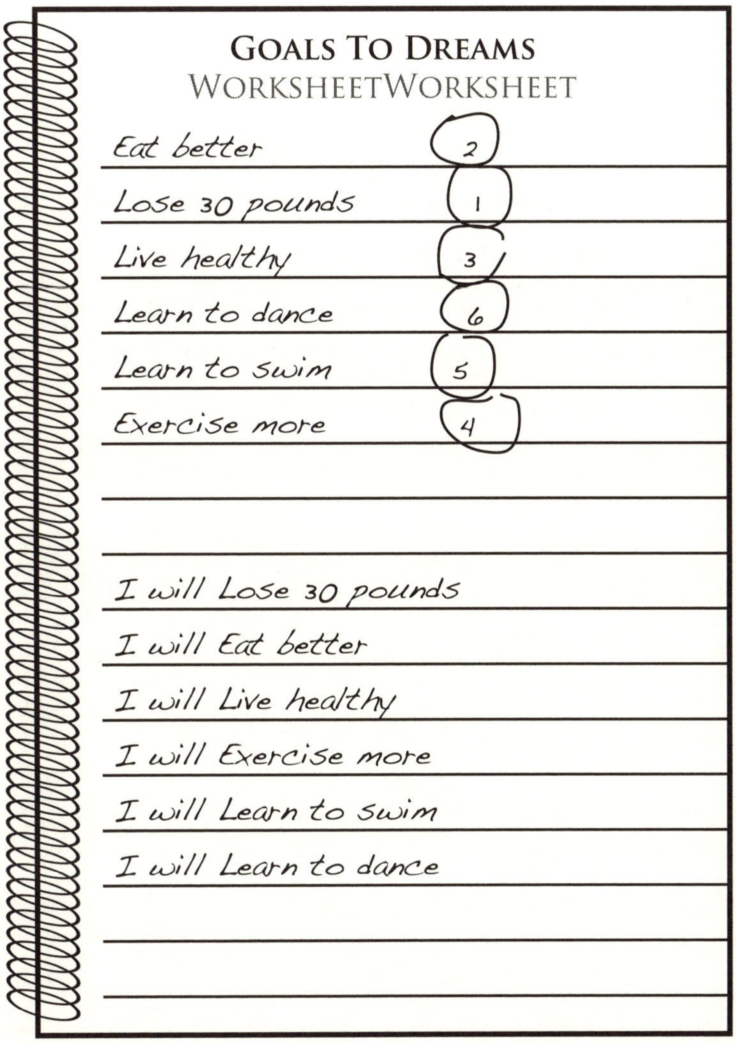

In the next chapter, you will learn what to do with this list and how it will become your itinerary to success. This list will help you complete more than you have ever thought you could. Find out how to use this list to your full advantage. If you haven't made your goal list yet, stop now, and do so before you continue reading.

"To move forward, you need to look forward."

"Success is not achieved by accident. Success is achieved by design."

SUMMARY

- The first step will often determine the level of success.
- Tracking and documenting your progress are required for success.
- Turn dreams into a goal list: document, prioritize, and quantify.
- The goal list that you created is your itinerary to success.

Chapter Eight

MAKING GOALS HAPPEN

Imagine if you could achieve any goal you set. You can and many people do just that. Every successful person sets goals. They include CEOs, business owners, managers, bodybuilders, teachers, salespeople, and anyone who excels in life and career. These people write down their goals, and they set a date or establish a timeline for accomplishing each one. Larger goals need to be broken down into subgoals, which are manageable, step-by-step approaches to the main goal. If this kind of goal setting is new to you, you'll be amazed at how powerful the process can be. See and appreciate the power of making goals. Refer to your goals often. If you don't record your goals, they will drift away like a warm summer breeze: it feels good while it is around, but when it is gone, you don't notice.

A goal is like an address; it's your destination. Can you imagine going to your friend's house for the first time and her directions are, "I live in California"? Will you find her house? How about if she says, "I live in Los Angeles"? You still would not find her house. What if she said, "I live on Main Street"? You might find her if you went house-to-house knocking on front doors. What if she told you, "I live at 24 Main Street. Take exit 4 and make a right on Main, and I am the eighth house on the left"? Now you can find her house without any trouble. Your goals need to be this precise. You must have the specific destination of your goal. Where do you want to go?

WISHES TO GOALS

You have decided which dreams are important, turned them into a goal list, and prioritized them. In this next step, you will determine whether your goals are realistic, and you will set a beginning and end for each goal. Suppose one of your goals is to lose 30 pounds. Is losing 30 pounds a realistic amount to lose? Look at the Body Mass Index (BMI) chart (page 216) and find your height on the vertical axis. Amy is a woman of average height, 5'4", and average frame type. She follows the line from 5'4" horizontally; it says that she should weigh between 108 pounds and 142 pounds, or between 18.5 BMI and 25 BMI respectively. Obviously, the closer that you are to the BMI of 25, the closer you are to being overweight. Also, consider your frame type. If you have a small frame, then you want a lower BMI. Conversely, if you have a large frame, you may be closer to a BMI of 25 and still be in excellent shape. The BMI chart is a rule of thumb for a person of average structure for that height category. A fit person should have low body fat, an active lifestyle, healthy dietary habits, and most important, a pleasant feeling about that reflection in the mirror. In the example, Amy, who is of medium frame, wants to be an average healthy weight, so her goal is halfway between 108 and 142, or 125 pounds. After stepping on a scale, she finds that she weighs 165.

165	Amy's current weight
- 125	The average fit weight for 5'4"
40	Number of pounds that Amy needs to lose to reach her goal

This means that if she wants to be an average fit weight of 125, she must lose 40 pounds instead of 30 pounds. After considering this information, she decides to lose 30 pounds for a final weight of 135 pounds, the same weight as when she graduated from high school. She decides that this is ambitious at this point. In her notebook, she can revise her goal to, "I will lose 30 pounds for a final weight of 135 pounds."

AT WHAT TIME?

If your friend did not tell you what time to come over for a visit, how would you know when to be there? Are you going for lunch or dinner? Are you planning to exercise together? If so, on what day and at what time? Without a time frame for reaching a goal, you will probably never get there. At work, if management didn't set deadlines for projects, would the projects ever be done? Wouldn't the coffee klatch or the water cooler conferences get in the way? Don't forget the day-to-day business errands and tasks.

Do you get the point? Without a prioritized timeline, life will throw a million reasons or "emergencies" at you and keep you from your goals. Interruptions and interferences happen every day to all of us. Why do you need to lose weight? Did you let body maintenance go by the wayside? Did life get in the way? People who are overweight have neglected body maintenance because it is not a priority. The body fat seems to sneak up quickly. One day you see yourself in a picture or the mirror and you ask yourself, "When did this happen?"

It's pointless to tell yourself, "One day I will be thin," or "One day I will lose weight." "One day" comments are unsuccessful comments! Most people know and say, "I *should* lose weight. I *should* exercise. I *should* eat better." When you do this, you *"should"* all over yourself. Goals need to be a "must." When you *must* lose 30 pounds, it will happen. When you *should* do something, it will never happen.

For you to be successful in any endeavor, your goals must have timelines. Goals are rarely unrealistic; they only have unreasonable time frames. For instance, to have a goal of losing 30 pounds in 1 month is unrealistic. To lose 30 pounds in 4 months is reasonable, achievable, and safe.

How can you know how long you will need to lose weight? Most physicians and experts agree that losing about 2 pounds a week is safe and realistic. That rate of weight loss offers the best chance of keeping weight off permanently. Amy wants to lose 30 pounds. That loss can safely be accomplished in 15 weeks. Thirty pounds divided by 2 pounds per week equals 15 weeks ($30 \div 2 = 15$). She can count out 15 weeks on the calendar, add 1 week for a margin of error, and then mark her calendar for her goal. When I set a goal, I also add it to my electronic calendar with periodic reminder notices that pop up on my computer screen as the date comes close.

When setting goals, you must set definitive targets and record them clearly. Without specific, definitive goals, you will flail and flounder in the face of adversity. However, with clearly defined goals, you can overcome any obstacle on your way toward victory. With a clear vision, your mind, body, and soul will be harmonized in one forward direction.

In addition to a time frame, goals must also have a starting point. This is a reference on which to base all subsequent comparisons. In other words, you must have a record of where you started so that you can measure your success and how far you have to go. In our example, Amy weighs 165 pounds. She will record this on the goal page of her journal. She will also record some basic body measurements, such as waist, hips, thighs, chest, arms, and BMI.

SIZE DOES MATTER!

At this point, your goals are set, but some are too large to be completed in one step. For example, to lose 30 pounds is an achievable goal, but it needs to be broken down into manageable pieces. Imagine if I did not create architectural plans and chart my goals and time frame before I started rehabilitating the old house. Could I have achieved the end result? No way! The old house needed a plan for framing, electricity, plumbing, wall board, and all of the other trades in a specific order and time frame. Your large goal needs to be segmented into subgoals or short-term goals. You will need a plan for exercise, muscle toning, nutrition, adversity, and scheduling.

Breaking down your main goals into subgoals will make them much easier to achieve. For example, imagine an 8-foot-tall wall in front of you. If reaching the top of that wall were your goal, how would you achieve it? You could jump, grab the edge, and maybe climb to the top, but that method is difficult or maybe even impossible for you. And every time you fell, you would be starting over from the same beginning point, looking up at that same 8-foot wall. What if you built a set of stairs to reach to the top of the wall? Wouldn't it be easier to walk to the top of the wall, one step at a time, on the staircase you built? You can now easily reach the top by working smarter, not harder. If you fall or stumble, you fall only one step. Such falls are easier to recover from, and you can continue on to your goal. The size of the goal does matter. If your goal is too big, it's a wall. You need a set of steps to get to the top.

Remember, we have determined that a safe and effective amount of weight to lose is 2 pounds a week, so Amy will write in her notebook, "I will lose 2 pounds a week for a final weight of 135." That is a good series of steps because she can monitor her progress weekly and adjust her methods if she is not making progress. In our example, Amy has set a date for her goal to be reached by counting out 16 weeks on her calendar. If you use that formula, you can easily set a goal date for weight loss. Other goals are just as easy to set. For instance, "to eat healthy foods" is a daily task, and it is a lifelong change to be implemented on a daily basis. Your goal should say, "I will eat healthy foods every day, making healthy choices most of the time."

It is time to let you in on an important weight management secret. If you are thinking, "It's impossible to eat healthy every day," you're right. I don't expect you to be perfect and neither should you. Expecting perfection destines you to failure. Instead, strive for excellence and progress. It is understandable that there will be days when you will not be able to abide by the rules: holidays, special events, engagements, and temporary lapses in good judgment happen to us all. You can, however, make the most appropriate decision for that day and most of the time. We will discuss this more fully in the "Nourishing Nutrition" section.

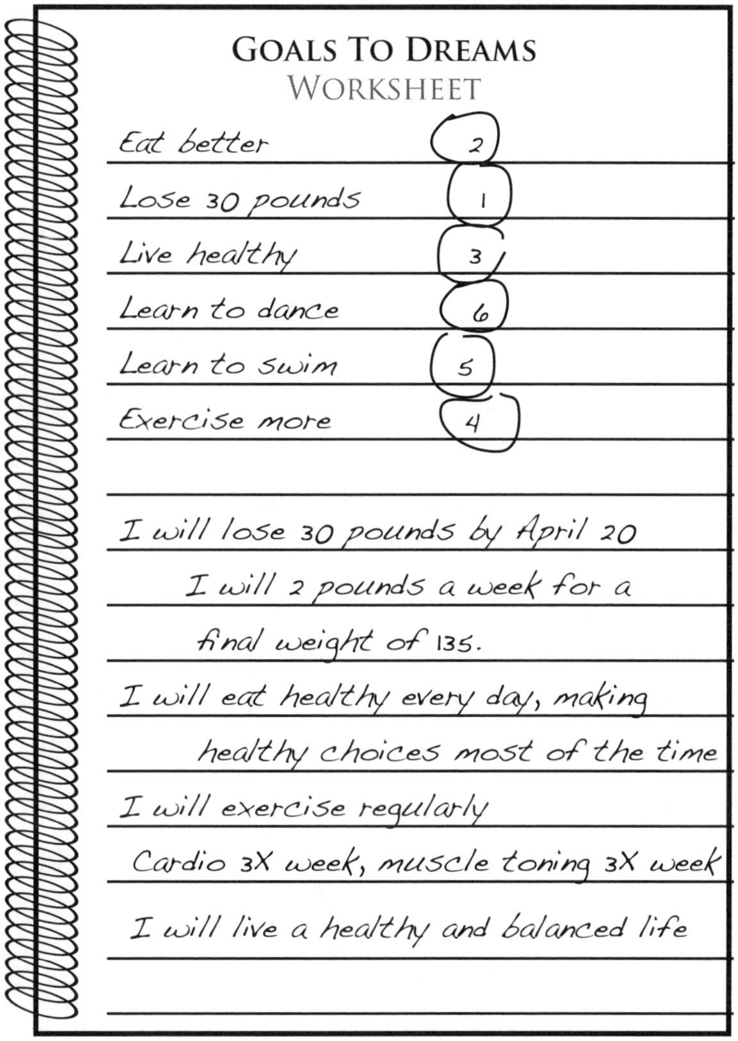

For the rest of this program, we will discuss

he first four goals illustrated in Amy's examples: to lose 30 pounds, to eat healthy foods, to live fit, and exercise regularly. I do encourage you to have other personal goals, such as learning to dance or swim, and to set a plan to achieve them. These are admirable goals and great avenues to self-development, not to mention that you'll have fun learning something new. My friends and I are always trying new things, taking classes to learn new skills, and continuing our education.

Open your *BetterBody BetterLife Journal* and complete your list of goals. Then turn to the next page, 54. You are now ready to make a permanent version of your completed list of goals from the second page. Copy your organized and developed goals from the second page to the first. This first page will now be a clean, crisp copy for reference. Remember, you can always add new goals or adjust your goals as required in the future.

"Faith is taking the first step even when you don't see the whole staircase."

-MARTIN LUTHER KING, JR.

SUMMARY

- Successful people set and document goals with a timeline.
- Set clear and definitive goals.
- Verify that goals are realistic and achievable.
- Goals are rarely unrealistic; they simply have unrealistic time frames.
- To reach the top of the wall, you must first build a staircase. You will climb to your goal more easily if you take many small, achievable steps.
- With a clear vision, your mind, body, and soul will move in harmony in one forward direction.
- Expecting perfection destines you to failure; instead, you should strive for excellence and progress.

MY STARTING POINT	
NAME	Amy
DATE	Jan 6
AGE	35
WEIGHT	165 lbs
HEIGHT	5'4"
BMI	30

MEASURMENTS	
WAIST	37"
HIPS	40"
CHEST	38.5/33.5"
THIGHS	24"
ARMS	14"
DRESS/PANT	12

DREAMS TO GOALS

I will lose 30 pounds by April 27 (16 weeks)

I will lose 2 pounds a week for a final weight of 135 lbs

I will eat healthy every day, making healthy choices most of the time.

I will exercise regularly

Cardio 3X week, Muscle toning 3X week

I will live a healthy and balanced life, striving to do better every day.

Amy

Chapter Nine

PLAN FOR SUCCESS

We're off to a great start. Can you feel the success building inside of you already? You have turned your dreams into goals, set realistic time frames for completion, and composed both your goals and your time frame in a positive, motivating, and achievable format. You have broken larger goals down into achievable subgoals, and you have determined what you will do. Now we will figure out how you are going to get to your goal. Becoming healthy and living well are not difficult when you break them down into day-by-day, event-by-event steps. The best chance of success comes from solid step-by-step strategies employed every day.

PLAN YOUR LIFE AND LIVE YOUR PLAN

I learned an important lesson when I became a scuba instructor. It's the diver's mantra: "Plan your dive and dive your plan." This philosophy keeps a diver safe in circumstances that could otherwise be dangerous. When participating in a sport that can be deadly if performed improperly, you must plan. Living your life improperly can be deadly, too. If you perform your life improperly and do not plan your life and health, the consequences will be debilitating medical issues and disease. Plan your life and live your plan.

DAILY MOTION

A great plan includes daily plans, short-term plans, long-term plans, and adversity plans. Every day you must keep your body in motion with day-by-day plans, or steps, to be achieved. Success is not a destination. Success is a journey. And journeys are made step-by-step.

For instance, if you want to learn a second language, you need to practice often, even daily, to become fluent. You will never become proficient in that language if you don't. I know this too well. I have been "trying" to learn another language for years without significant progress because I do not have a plan and do not practice regularly. The same is true with your body. How long have you been "trying" to lose weight? If you practice — that is, work at the plan every day — you will come closer to obtaining your goals with each day. You will experience small but consistent change. This is the plan to achieve permanent weight loss; there is no other successful method.

ADVERSITY PLANS

To achieve your weight-loss goals, you must have adversity plans. They will help you stay on track when situations arise that would normally lead you astray. If you have a chronic issue with snacking, then you should have an adversity plan that minimizes unproductive snacking. That plan may be to have something healthful ready and available to eat, or you may plan an activity to occupy your mind. The best adversity plan is to do something that raises your heart rate and changes your physiology, such as taking a short, brisk walk or stretching your muscles at your desk. Such activities take only a minute or two, and you'll be rewarded with a great rush from the blood flowing through your arteries.

You must also plan for forgiveness. We all need to permit ourselves some devilish treats at times. I have unhealthful foods at times, and you can, too — but only occasionally and in moderation. The occasional treat is perfectly acceptable— in fact, even necessary. It is important to learn when it is okay to say yes to foods and activities that do not promote your goals. If, however, you find that you are having too many detrimental treats or are lounging on the couch too often, you will know that you need to make adjustments in your plan.

Everyone falls prey to urges or displays a temporary lack of good judgment. It is part of being human. To be successful you need to learn from these events and learn how to minimize setbacks in the future. With each failure comes an opportunity for a future success. There is no shame in falling off course, only in staying off course. Don't expect perfection; it doesn't exist.

Strive for the exceptional and never stop moving forward. If you fail at your plan one day, analyze the reasons why you faltered. Your analysis will teach you how to defeat the urge the next day. Success is moving forward more than you fall back. Success is establishing a goal and working until you achieve it. Success means never stopping trying. Read this paragraph again. It is essential in life.

FOR THE RECORD

To help you move toward your goals, record events, efforts, and weaknesses throughout the day. At the end of each day, review your daily journal. Analyze the day's efforts and figure out what to do better the next day. This kind of review is an essential part of your plan. If you are not doing this now, you should start. It is a profound way to become a greater person and achieve goals, especially if you are completely honest with yourself. (See journal example on the next page.)

The *BetterBody BetterLife Journal* will help you make progress toward your fitness and weight-loss goals. You can use it to track and evaluate your efforts. After you have reviewed the day and evaluated your progress, immediately plan for the next day. Decide what you will eat at each meal and make a plan to handle adversity. Decide what you will do when cravings come or when your schedule is disrupted. For example, if you know that you get cravings in the afternoon, plan an event to take the place of snacking. Take a walk, drink a glass of water, knock something off the to-do-list, or eat a healthful treat (planned and ready) instead of surrendering to the vending machine urge that you will regret later.

The purpose is to replace the subconscious habit, a learned behavior of unplanned snacking, with a productive habit. This is particularly helpful if the snacking is induced by a powerful emotion such as boredom or sadness. By planning and employing the eating techniques that you will learn in the "*Nourishing Nutrition*" section, you can conquer any adversity. You can also plan ahead for your exercise routine. If you know that you usually do not have the time or the energy to exercise at the end of the day, then plan to exercise first thing in the morning or at some other time that is convenient and consistent. As you evaluate your day, evaluate the quality of your exercise routine. Was the workout good or bad? Did you miss it altogether? If it was not a great workout, you can figure out why and then try to make changes to promote a great workout.

MUSCLE TONING

UPPER BODY - Chest, Shoulders, & Arms

Planned Start Time 7:00 am Actual Start Time 7:15 am

Planned Exercise				Actual Exercise			
Exercise	Reps	Resistance	Minutes Rest	Exercise	Reps	Resistance	Minutes Rest
CHEST							
Chest Press	20	50%	1	Dumbbell Press	20	10 lbs	1
Chest Press	12	80%	1	Dumbbell Press	12	15 lbs	1
Chest Press	12	100%	1	Dumbbell Press	12	20 lbs	1
Pec Flyes	12	100%	1	Dumbbell pec flyes	12	15 each	1
Pec Flyes	12	100%	1	Dumbbell pec flyes	12	15 lbs	1
SHOULDERS							
Shoulder Press	12	100%	1	Shoulder Press	12	20 lbs	1
Shoulder Press	12	100%	1	Shoulder Press	12	20 lbs	1
Lateral Raises	12	100%	1	Lateral Raises	12	15 lbs	1
Lateral Raises	12	100%	1	Lateral Raises	12	15 lbs	1
BICEPS							
Dumbbell Curls	12	100%	1	Dumbbell Curls	12	20 lbs	1
Dumbbell Curls	12	100%	1	Dumbbell Curls	12	20 lbs	1
Dumbbell Curls	12	100%	1	Dumbbell Curls	12	20 lbs	1
TRICEPS							
Tri Extensions	12	100%	1	Tri Ext	12	20 lbs	1
Tri Extensions	12	100%	1	Tri Ext	12	20 lbs	1
Tri Pull-Downs	12	100%	1	Tri Pull-Downs	12	20 lbs	1

Note: Exercises filled in gray are suggested. Fill in the exercise that you choose to do.

Note: Resistance column is the weight used or the resistance number.

Notes: This was a great day! I worked out in the a.m. and finished strong. I felt so good for the rest of the day. I was a little sore, but it is a good sore. Next time I need to increase my weights for tricep exercises. I also need to drink more water during the work-out. I must start by 7am so my morning is not rushed. A++ day!

In your planning, consider the special events that are a part of your calendar. Plan your meals and fitness routine simultaneously to avoid conflicts. For instance, if you know that you will be going out to dinner and that you will want to indulge in a magnificent dessert, you may also decide to make this your day off and not be concerned with your food choices. Or you may complete your fitness routine in the morning and adjust the amount of fat and calories (energy) you consume during the day to help compensate for the dessert. Don't, however, skip meals. You'll get so hungry you may end up eating twice what you should.

This kind of planning and evaluating may sound like a lot to do each night, but it takes fewer than 10 minutes to evaluate one day and plan for the next. The whole *BetterBody BetterLife* program takes less than 3 percent of your day, including the planning and evaluating: 30 minutes for your fitness routine and 10 minutes for planning and analyzing your progress. Every step is important. In time the process will become second nature, and you'll need to expend only a little effort to get results that last a lifetime.

Will you have to keep a record of everything you do for the rest of your life? No. In time healthy living will become natural and instinctive. But you should keep your journal faithfully until you have reached your weight and fitness goals; then continue until you have determined the right maintenance plan for you. For some people, this determination may take only 3 or 4 months; others may need 2 or 3 years. Some choose to keep this routine as a permanent part of their life because it promotes fitness management.

Are you resistant to the idea of recording and planning? Consider this: You have lived with excess body fat for a long time, most likely years or even decades, and you've probably tried numerous diets to lose the weight. Have you been successful yet? Your journal is a key tool for your success. A few minutes a day with it will help assure that you reach your health and fitness goals. I recommend that you use this tool for the rest of your life. It will help you reach all your goals.

THE SUBCONSCIOUS

Each night before you retire, look at your goal page and recite your list to yourself. Say it out loud. Repetition will plant the seed of success. Every night while you sleep, your mind processes what you have experienced and learned the day before. Make your goals the first and last thought of every day so that your other-than-conscious brain can process and assimilate those goals. What you think about most — you become. You should also review your goals when you are lacking motivation. Your list may not motivate you instantly, but it will incubate in your mind and create motivation. Make a copy of your goals list and keep it with you for reference and inspiration.

After a period of time, your goals will naturally be foremost in your mind. You will not have to think about them because they will become a part of you. How many times have you gone to work without putting your clothes on? "Hey Amy! You forgot something again!" It never happens. You instinctively get dressed before you leave the house each day. Healthy living will enter your subconscious in that same way. Your goals will become part of your internal code; they will become part of your thoughts and emotions. Instinctively, you will make the best choices most of the time. If you are about to order a bacon cheeseburger with large fries, you will get a funny feeling in your gut. No, it is not your stomach saying, "No, not again!" But it might be. When you get that feeling, you will be forced to decide consciously if you are making an appropriate choice. Instead of feeling guilty with eater's remorse after eating your meal, you will have the opportunity and the power to decide if that meal is allowable and acceptable to your goals.

All successful people take account of the efficiency and productivity of each day. They analyze each event and look for opportunities to improve. Do the same and you will be successful at weight loss and fitness management. I have a friend who uses an effective method of self-improvement; it is the main reason for his distinguished success. Once a week, he goes into his home office to review his day planner with his notes from the week. He mentally reviews the meetings, conversations, and events of the last 7 days. He asks himself, "What did I do wrong? What can I improve? How can I improve? What did I do right, and how can I repeat my successes to improve my performance? What lessons have I learned?" At the start, he found this exercise a bit distressing, but in time, he found that he made fewer mistakes. He identified areas for improvement and praised himself for his successes.

Review your day each evening. Analyze your choices and look for ways to improve yourself. Find pitfalls and figure out what you can do to eliminate them. Most important, focus on the successes you had throughout the day and then pat yourself on the back so you will repeat those successes in the future. You will then sleep well knowing you are succeeding and moving toward your goals.

PROCRASTINATION

Procrastination is the evil of all evils. It can make even the strongest people fall short of their goals. Second to a lack of planning, it is the most common reason for failure. How do successful people overcome procrastination? They form a plan for each day, they set a number of items to accomplish, and they do not stop until each one is done. You will not find CEOs sitting on the couch watching television for hours at a time, nor will you will find a doctor sleeping until noon on the weekends. They are always moving toward their goals, which is why they are so successful.

It is easy to procrastinate. If you know you have a problem with your roof, you tell yourself that you will call the roofer in the morning. The next morning comes around and you rush to get the kids to school on time. Then you forget to call the roofer the following day and the day after that. Weeks go by and a storm rolls in. The rain leaks into your home, ruining the ceiling and the walls and a treasured family portrait. Oh, no! Every roofer you call says that he can't make it for weeks because of other "emergencies." In the weeks that follow, rain falls every day and causes more damage to your home. The previous owners of my house across from Joe's Corner Store let decades go by, procrastinating and neglecting the old house to the point of structural failure. Do you know someone who has done the same thing to his or her body? Have you?

This is what happens to most people and their bodies. Maintenance is put off until one day an emergency arises, and a crash diet is thought to be in order. Unfortunately, crash diets don't work, and the yo-yo cycle begins. Stop neglecting your body and make the changes that produce permanent results. Sitting on the couch does little for your mind and nothing for your body. If you catch yourself in front of the tube, especially if you are flipping the channels mindlessly, turn the TV off and do something productive. Go for a walk, take out the trash, read a book, or go kiss your spouse. Play with your children or the dog; take care of the projects on your to-do-list. A body in motion will stay in motion, with little effort to do so. A body that is sedentary is likely to stay sedentary, growing weak and ill.

"To reach a destination you must start with the first step, then continue to place one foot in front of the other."

SUMMARY

- Plan your life and live your plan.
- To be successful you must plan every day.
- Make adversity plans to conquer your weaknesses.
- Plan for allowance and forgiveness.
- Review and evaluate your efforts each day.
- If you falter, evaluate the reason and plan better.
- Never stop improving!
- Each night and morning, review your goal page. Allow your goals to enter your subconscious.
- Procrastination is the opposite of success.

Chapter Ten

LIGHTS, CAMERA, ACTION!

We tend to see ourselves the way we wish to be. The distortion can be small or large. This chapter is about looking at yourself from a different perspective, from other people's perspective. It is important to document your starting point with irrefutable evidence. This step may surprise and enlighten you. It will give you a reference of where you started and reinforce why you are learning to live healthily and lose weight. If you wander and need direction, you can refer back to this step and ask yourself, "Do I want to go back to being like that?"

To gain insight into your physical condition, you need to see yourself through the eyes of others. This unquestionable and unbiased proof comes in the form of a photograph. To obtain the proof, you need your camera. Don't panic! This is for your reference only. Do not detour around this; it is a critical step in your progress. This step alone is all the motivation that some people need.

You will accomplish three objectives in this step:
First: You will create a reference tool and a record of where you started. This tool will help determine how far you need to go.

Second: You will see how others see you. Sometimes mirrors lie (actually the perception of what you see), but pictures show the world as we all see it. (No trick photography allowed.)

Third: A picture will help you look at yourself objectively. This is not a self-bashing opportunity, but a self-improvement opportunity.

STOP THE DISTRACTIONS

The best place to take your pictures is in front of a plain wall or simple background. Allow no distractions behind you in the photo. Choose a supportive person to take your pictures, perhaps a friend or relative who is in the *BetterBody BetterLife* program with you. Some highly determined people go as far as hiring a professional to take the pictures. You can also use a tripod and a camera with a timer if you have them.

Women should wear a swimsuit, and men should wear snug shorts. You want to see your body, not the clothes that you are wearing. The purpose of taking pictures is to show your entire figure. Face the camera and stand in a normal manner; do not slouch or stand too erect. Do not suck your belly in or push it out. Just stand in an everyday way. Take three pictures of your front. Next, face away from the camera and take three pictures of your backside. Last, take two profile pictures (side views) of each side. Remember to stand in your normal manner. You should now have a total of ten pictures of yourself from four different angles. Now take pictures of your partner who is doing the *BetterBody BetterLife* plan with you. Drop the film off to be developed or print the pictures yourself if you are using a digital camera and printer.

DON'T GET CAUGHT OFF GUARD

Do you look different than you thought you would? I have found that many people are shocked at the condition of their bodies. "I knew I was carrying a few extra pounds, but I didn't expect to look like this!" This is your reality check. Seeing these pictures might be enough in itself to prompt you to make the commitment to get fit. It was for me. Don't get caught off guard as I was. I was on a scuba diving trip as a volunteer for a nonprofit marine research organization. Every event was photographed throughout the week. A few months later, I was looking through the new issue of a scuba-diving magazine, and I found an article about our trip. I was surprised to find it, and I read it enthusiastically. I studied the photos, but could not identify the person who was wearing shorts and no shirt. I thought, *That can't be me; he's too stocky.* Then I recognized my watch and cap. I was horrified. I couldn't recognize myself. My friends even said, "Is that you? Those love handles offer a large grip!" I was thankful that I didn't see a caption with my name! Do you have to see yourself in an international magazine to make a change?

This step is important because the best way to see yourself is through the lens of a camera. Your long-term progress will be greater than your short-term embarrassment. As you look at the photos, pick one picture of each view. Use the ones that have the best focus and color. Paste the pictures in your journal, saving the best photo (front view) for the "Picture Plaque," which we will discuss in the next chapter.

"Whatever the mind can conceive and believe, it can achieve."

NAPOLEON HILL, AUTHOR

SUMMARY

- See yourself as the world sees you.
- Your photographs are a record of your starting point.
- Use your photos for motivation.
- When reviewing your photos, look at yourself objectively.
- No self-bashing!

Chapter Eleven

GOT MOTIVATION?

How do you get motivated and stay motivated? Without inspiration and motivation, very few people succeed or even get started. This chapter will teach you methods and give you tools for getting and staying motivated. Everything that you do is the result of motivation. You go to work to earn money to keep a roof over your head. You eat to keep from starving, and you are affectionate when you want affection in return. Everything is the result of a motive to solve a problem, or — in the language I prefer — to meet a challenge. You are reading this book because you have a challenge in health and fitness, as I once did.

I want to live a long, healthy, and robust life and to help others do the same. Those desires motivate me to learn everything I can about health and fitness. And I never stop learning. I continue my education at intensive weekend courses for that purpose. Learning new and better ways to live keeps me jazzed. You should be so excited to start your new life that you are overflowing with anticipation. I have lived my life with an exuberant attitude, and I want you to feel that with me. When you get into better shape and liberate yourself from excess weight, you will feel that exuberance every day. I love life. I want to be here for a very long time with a very active lifestyle, and I want you to be here with me. This is why I live the way that I do and why I created the *BetterBody BetterLife* program.

Before we discuss how to motivate ourselves, we should define *motivate.* According to *Webster's New World Dictionary* the verb *motivate* means "to provide with, or affect as, a motive; incite." Incite means to urge to action. A motive is an inner drive, an impulse that causes one to act.

Motivation comes from within you. It must be in your gut, in your heart, or in your soul. It needs to be a fire that will not be extinguished. My core motivation, the one that is deep within my soul and that keeps me living healthily every day, is that I know the consequences if I do not take care of myself. I see the pain and the suffering that so many bear because they are overweight. I am willing to work to avoid an old age crippled by medical issues and a retirement highlighted by doctors' visits and a move to a nursing home. I know that if I invest a little time in health each day, I improve my chances of living a life that is full and active at every age. I want the same for you.

How many relatives and friends have you seen wither away from poor health? Who among those close to you are overweight and missing out on life? How many relatives and friends have you seen pass away before their time because of cardiac complications? How long have you been putting off a healthy lifestyle by saying, "I will do it tomorrow, next week, next month, or next year?" How long will you keep waiting?

I was reminded of how much body fat I have lost when I took my 18-month-old daughter to her pediatrician for a physical. Her weight in pounds is very nearly equal to what I lost. When I held her, I weighed the same as I once did. I used to carry that extra weight every hour of every day. It slowed me down, made me fatigued, and stressed out my organs. I notice a marked difference in my sleep and my brain function since I lost the weight. I have more energy and endurance, plus my clothes always fit because I am a constant and steady weight. I don't have to worry about buying an expensive outfit because I know it will fit me until it wears out. It is truly phenomenal. It is fun when I meet someone I haven't seen in 10 or 20 years and I still look as fit as I did in high school. How much "baby fat" are you wearing?

Motivations are as different as people are, so while reading the next few pages, consider what excites you most and what scares you most. Customize the framework that I show you. Everyone has different reasons and references for motivation. Some are motivated by the thought of clogged arteries, other by a lack of physical energy, and others by the thought that they may not be around to see their children or grandchildren graduate from college. Whatever your motivation, remind yourself of the pain you face if you do not follow through. Imagine your daughter getting married without her mom as mother-of-the-bride. Imagine lying in a hospital bed about to be put under anesthesia for open-heart surgery. Imagine all the vacations you have worked hard to earn all your life but cannot take because of medical issues. How will you feel when your medical bills *eat* your retirement nest egg? It is this pain that will get you through those days when you do not feel like exercising or when you need incentive to make the right food choice.

Our primary human needs are to avoid pain and to gain pleasure. For many people, food gives pleasure and diminishes pain. We eat out of habit, but we also eat to escape temporarily from the pain of boredom, social anxiety, and depression. Food can make you feel good in the moment, and can be an easy, quick fix to a bigger problem. For some people, the fear of failing on another diet is more painful than trying another diet. (Good thing this is not a diet.) Many people associate pain with fitness and health because they have spent a lifetime with poor health habits and the unknowns of healthy living are scary. Perhaps you have been living an unhealthy lifestyle for years, maybe even decades. Change means you will leave that lifestyle behind. Although you know that the life you wish for is a better life, you learned to be comfortable in your current life.

The truth is that it is more painful to stay overweight than it is to do something about it. You know that is true, don't you? You know you must do something about your weight, don't you? It is up to you and only you. You must create your life. You can create your life. Sometimes that is easier said than done. This challenge can be overcome with leverage. You can leverage yourself past your fears, past your current habits, and past the beliefs that are keeping you in an unhealthy lifestyle. The best way to do that is with an exercise. Read the following four paragraphs; then sit back and do the exercise.

> Imagine that you started a healthy lifestyle change 5 years ago. You would be healthy and fit right now. You would be doing things you are not doing today because your weight or health problems are holding you back. How great would life be now? You would be buying clothes off the rack and looking wonderful. Maybe you would

be going on vacations and doing everything you want from dawn to late night. You would be feeling great, sleeping well, and looking good.

Now, imagine 5 years in the future. What will you be like if you do NOT start healthy living now? Will you be in the same circumstances you are now? Will you be worse? I am not projecting this on you, but the following happens to most people: Your habits get worse, you gain more weight, and you end up in worse condition. You will still be fighting the battle with diets, or maybe you will have given up. You may believe that being fat is your destiny. You will not like what you see in the mirror or how you feel about your physical condition.

Now imagine 10 years in the future if you still have not started healthy living. You will be fatter and sicker. You will feel even worse about yourself. Your body will have deteriorated extensively, and your major physiological systems will not be functioning well. Your liver, kidneys, and heart will be working overtime. Even worse, will you even be here in 10 years if you continue to live the same way you are now? What about in 15 years or 20? What will your health be then?

Stop now, sit in a quiet area and close your eyes and think about what your life will be like if you do not start living a healthy lifestyle now. What will you look like? How will you feel? How many doctors' visits will you have for health problems? How much will you regret not changing your life today — at this very moment? Close your eyes and imagine your future if you do not change.

Did you do the exercise? If not, do it...please.

This is a sobering exercise to help you gain insight into your potential future. The exercise is not meant to lead you to pity yourself or feel bad about your past, but to gain leverage. It should help you comprehend the pain you will feel if you do not make a change. Nearly two-thirds of Americans are overweight or obese. If you continue to live like the masses with junk food, fast food, processed food, and being a couch potato, you — like the masses — will be fat for the rest of your life. Just because the masses live in a certain way does not make their actions right. Not too long ago, many

Americans smoked and thought smoking was cool. There were no health warnings about it, and it was socially acceptable. Now the health issues of smoking are well known, and far fewer people smoke.

Looking back, we all have made choices that we wish we hadn't. Most of the time, we are making the best choices that we can with the knowledge and experience that we have at that moment. Please do not be the one who looks back 10 years from now and says, "I should have started a decade ago when I read that book." From this program, you will gain the knowledge that you need to adopt a healthy lifestyle and lose weight without dieting. Those things will happen only if you are willing. Nobody can help you if you are not willing. Nobody can make you live any differently than you are now, except you. Make the change for the beautiful person you are; do it for yourself. You are an amazing and exceptional person, and you can achieve anything you set your heart to. Your family and loved ones will be grateful; you will be an example, and they will learn from your successes.

Are you afraid that becoming fit and healthy will change your relationships? Such a concern may sound silly, but many people fear that if they become healthy, their friends and family will envy them or dislike their new lifestyle. They worry that weight loss may mean missing out on special times with family or friends, such as social gatherings over big meals or meetings at the Cheesecake Factory. First, if you need food as a social lubricant, then you need to get a life or get new friends. What you have in common and admire about each other should be the bond, not food. Second, this fear is unfounded. My dietary habits are very different from some of my buddies, but they haven't gotten in the way of our having a good time. Sometimes I get teased about my meal as my friends scarf down their third dozen of Buffalo wings (the way I used to eat). They are not laughing when I can run circles around them on the court. They are not laughing as they complain about the spare tires they cannot seem to get rid of.

Instead of worrying, hope that when you transform your body, others will follow your example. You can be a motivation for others to lose weight and live healthily. You can be the one people talk about when they say, "If she can do it, I can do it!"

After avoiding pain, the other primary human need is to receive pleasure. We all like to receive pleasure, but we do not always choose a positive pleasure. Unfortunately, many people opt for the short-term "perceived" pleasure instead of the long-term "true" pleasure. This is why drug addicts have such a hard time kicking their addiction. The drug gives them instant gratification, a quick fix. Once the high wears off, they need another hit.

Instant gratification is also the reason why so many people are overweight. The short-term pleasure of a pint of ice cream is chosen over the long-term pleasure of eating something healthy. When the guilt settles in from eating the ice cream, another event must happen to induce pleasure again. It is likely that event will be food again. This can be a vicious cycle. The key is to recognize the pattern and stop it. If you choose a true long-term pleasure such as regular exercise, you live on a natural high that doesn't wear off.

The remainder of this chapter offers tools and techniques for staying motivated and achieving long-term pleasure. Do you want to feel like a million bucks? Then get your body running like a million-dollar machine. If you do, you will look like a million bucks, too. Imagine how much fun you will have shopping and buying new, smaller clothes. Think about how wonderful you will feel when your friends compliment you because you look healthy and happy. Your plans for staying motivated must be very personal; they should arise from your pleasure motivations, not from someone else's idea of a reward or what someone else thinks you should do.

YOUR TOOLS

Pictures and photographs of what you want to achieve are important motivational tools. You might choose a picture of someone with the physique of a fitness instructor or a photograph of you when you were younger and in better condition. Perhaps a picture of a full-figured model who is smaller than you or more toned will help you. The key is to use something that is realistic for you and consistent with the goals that you outlined for yourself in the previous chapters. If you are 6 feet tall with a large frame, a picture of a petite model is not very helpful, just as a woman who is 5 feet tall should not use pictures of a 5'10" runway model. There are many people out there whose size and body type are similar to yours. Magazines are usually the best places to look for pictures. Don't forget product advertisements featuring ordinary people. The person you select does not have to be famous. The important thing is that the pictures should be realistic for you; they should illustrate what you want to look like. This picture will be used to represent your goal in the "Picture Plaque" on the next page.

AN INSPIRATIONAL TOOL

You also need a picture of something that you want, but can't have, because of your weight or poor health. Your picture might show an outfit that you would love to wear, or you might choose a brochure of a Disney World vacation that you would love to take, but can't because you are not fit enough for the extensive walking the trip requires. Your inspirational picture could show a public pool or beach where you are too embarrassed to go because of your appearance in a bathing suit.

Such pictures will help you stay on track throughout the next several months. Take the three or four pictures that best exhibit what you want to achieve and tape them in a prominent place, perhaps on your bathroom mirror or in the area where you get dressed in the morning. A picture on the door of the fridge will be a great reminder and incentive each time you go to find some food for a meal or snack. The picture does not have to be in a place where your friends or family can see it, but it must be in a place where you will see it and recall every day what you want to accomplish. When you see the picture, you will be reminded of your goals, and you'll remember to make appropriate decisions throughout the day. Your inspirational pictures will change as you achieve your goals, but don't take the old ones down. Replace them with new inspirational pictures.

THE PICTURE PLAQUE

Your weight-loss plan will probably require more than one goal picture. Just as you broke down your goals into subgoals, your pictures need to reflect different stages of your quest. If your goal is to lose 30 pounds, then you need more than one picture. You need three or four pictures to visualize your goal. If you do not break your larger goal down into subgoals, you'll feel as if you need an eternity to reach your goal. Multiple goals are motivating. Every time you attain a subgoal, your motivation will be renewed. Losing 10 pounds three times is easier than attaining one goal of 30 pounds. This way of thinking will work for any weight goal; simply change the numbers to coincide with your goals.

To make the goal-setting process easy for you, I will send you a "Picture Plaque" free if you go to www.BetterBodyBetterLife.com and click on "Picture Plaque." It has four spaces for pictures. In the first space, put a current photo of yourself, perhaps one facing forward toward the camera. Leave the next two spaces blank. In the last space put the picture that represents your goal.

In Amy's example, she wants to lose 30 pounds, so in the second position she writes, "I will lose 10 pounds," and on the next place, "I will lose 20 pounds." That is her goal divided by three. As she progresses and reaches each subgoal, she will paste new pictures of herself in the appropriate places. When Amy has lost 10 pounds, she will take a new picture of herself and tape it over the space that says, "I will lose 10 pounds." When she has lost another 10 pounds for a total weight loss of 20 pounds, she will take a new picture of herself at the new weight and tape it over the space labeled, "I will lose 20 pounds." When she has reached her ultimate goal of 30 pounds, she will take a new picture of herself and tape it over the picture that has represented her goal up until that point. If she picked an appropriate goal picture, she will look similar in physique to that person. Amy now has solid proof of what she has accomplished. You can do the same. Like Amy, you will be proud. You will want to show off the before, during, and after pictures of yourself. You are allowed to gloat, brag, and toot your own horn because you have accomplished so much.

BETTERBODY BETTERLIFE

PICTURE PLAQUE

Before Picture Goes Here	I Will Lose 10 Pounds	I Will Lose 20 Pounds	Goal Picture Goes Here

Let's imagine that you need to get from your home to the market in the dark of the night, and you do not turn on your headlights. Will you get there? Driving laws aside, you might make it if you drive slowly, but your trip will take much longer, and your chances for failure will be much greater. Your odds of a catastrophe are greater, too. Don't get left in the dark. Your pictures are your headlights. Let them help you see where you are starting and get to where you want to go.

You Need the Hype

Every morning when you wake up, look at your goal pictures and say to them, "I will look like you! That's gonna be me! I will get closer today!" YELL at 'em! Yes, I said yell at the pictures; then look yourself in the mirror and shout, "I CAN do it! I WILL do it! That WILL be me!" Not everyone can yell at the mirror and at a picture, but you can talk to them. Say those things out loud and mean them! Vocalizing your goals is an effective reinforcement tool. Speaking ingrains the thought into your conscious and subconscious. Give yelling a try; you might be amazed at how good it feels. You don't have to yell loudly; you don't want the neighbors thinking that you are in trouble. But then again, if you stay with your same sedentary, unhealthy lifestyle, you will be in trouble. When you look at your pictures, talk to yourself as if you were a commander — forceful, brisk, and in control. Command yourself to achieve your goals. Most important, get excited!

I have three pictures that are an inspiration for me taped on my bathroom mirror. I have pictures inside the door to my closet and on the fridge. I keep fitness magazines all over the house — in the living room, in the bathrooms, on the nightstand, and in the kitchen. I find myself flipping through the pages as I cook, prepare for bed, or eat breakfast. When I lose momentum, I look at them, and then I look at myself in the mirror. This brings my goals to the forefront of my mind. If I do not feel like exercising, I look at a magazine and flip through it. I then remember why I set my goals, and I get inspired. I think of what I want to look like strolling on the beach or walking down the street in summer clothing. I often think of one of my pictures while I am exercising, cooking, or shopping for food. If my motivation wanes, I think of what life will be like in 20 years if I do not invest a little time in my fitness each day.

Other Tools

Magazines are great motivational tools. Go out and buy a few magazines to inspire you and then subscribe to those you like. Your favorite magazines could be about fitness, outdoor recreation, running, mountain biking, or even travel. Magazines provide a ready supply of motivational pictures and articles. Every time they arrive, they remind you of your goals. If the speed of life puts you on a detour, their reminders will help you get back on course. Furthermore, the new information in each issue will increase your knowledge. Remember, never stop learning.

That's What Friends Are For

A friend or partner is a great motivational tool. You don't have to have a fitness partner, but having one makes staying motivated easier and more fun. Your partner needs to have goals similar to yours. You don't have to be at the same level, but you do have to be going in the same direction — the direction of being fit and healthy.

Let's look at two of my friends as examples. He works out of their apartment, and she works long hours in an office. They rarely exercise together, but they still provide motivational support for each other. They even have very different goals, but they are going in the same direction. He wants to lose body fat and add 20 pounds of lean muscle. She wants to tone her body and lose 15 pounds. Here is how their partnership works: He goes to the gym to exercise in the morning, usually very early. She exercises during lunch at the gym in her office building. Sometimes, they go jogging or mountain biking together on a weekend. She takes her lunch with her; that way she gets her nutritional requirements in an appropriate meal during the workday. He eats at home and has the fridge stocked for him. At the end of the day, he typically cooks for them and has dinner ready when she gets home. They e-mail each other during the day or speak on the phone, asking about each other's workout. This communication is great because if one is unmotivated, hearing about the other's workout usually triggers the craving for a workout. This partnership works well for them because they both want to be lean, healthy, and energetic.

Although such a close partnership is ideal, you don't have to have someone to go step-by-step with you. You can even have a partner who is halfway across the country. By e-mail or by talking several times a week, you can help ensure each other's success. I coach people from around the country through e-mail and on the telephone. It works. When you talk, ask about each other's meals and workouts. Discuss each other's uncertainties and focus on each other's progress. You can give each other tips and techniques to overcome obstacles. This support will create motivation. It might even cause a little competition, which is even more motivating. You can discuss new recipes, workouts, or even new motivational tactics. Both of you can provide support and recognition — each for the other. You can even send updated photos to each other by e-mail.

When your partner goes down one dress size, you will be happy and more determined to keep up with her. If your partner loses another inch on her waist or thighs, you will want to try harder to achieve your goals. Of course, you and your partner might be at very different levels, and you must remember the difference when you compare your achievements to hers. Different people obtain different results at different rates. If you are not losing weight as fast as your friend, don't get discouraged. The most important thing is moving in the right direction, with both of you constantly reinforcing and praising each other. Success is continuing to make progress, so remember to help your partner attain her goals.

Motivation is, by definition, what makes you do everything that you do. Everything! Move from the body and lifestyle that you have now to the body and lifestyle that you want, using the motivational tools that work best for you. Some days will be tough, and you may want to give up or be lazy. On those days find motivation wherever you can. Call a friend, look in a magazine, or watch a fitness video; do whatever will change your state of mind. We have all been there; you are not alone. Everyone loses motivation, but winners find ways to get it back. We all have to overcome our obstacles and face our individual challenges. The path to success lies in finding what works for you, finding the motivational tools that inspire you. You must never give up! If you fall off course, adjust and get back on course. Remember: there is no shame in falling off course, only in staying off course. Simple actions can cause massive results. The results are a *better body* and a *better life*, a healthy life with more energy and a lot longer time on this planet to enjoy it.

"Success is not a destination but a journey."

SUMMARY

- Imagine 10 years in the future. What is your life like?
- You must want to change; the desire must come from within.
- Our primary human needs are avoiding pain and receiving pleasure.
- Get excited about every day and every success.
- Use inspirational tools. Find what motivates you.
- Use the "Picture Plaque" and post motivational photos everywhere.
- Use magazines as periodic reminders and motivation.
- Partners are a great motivation.

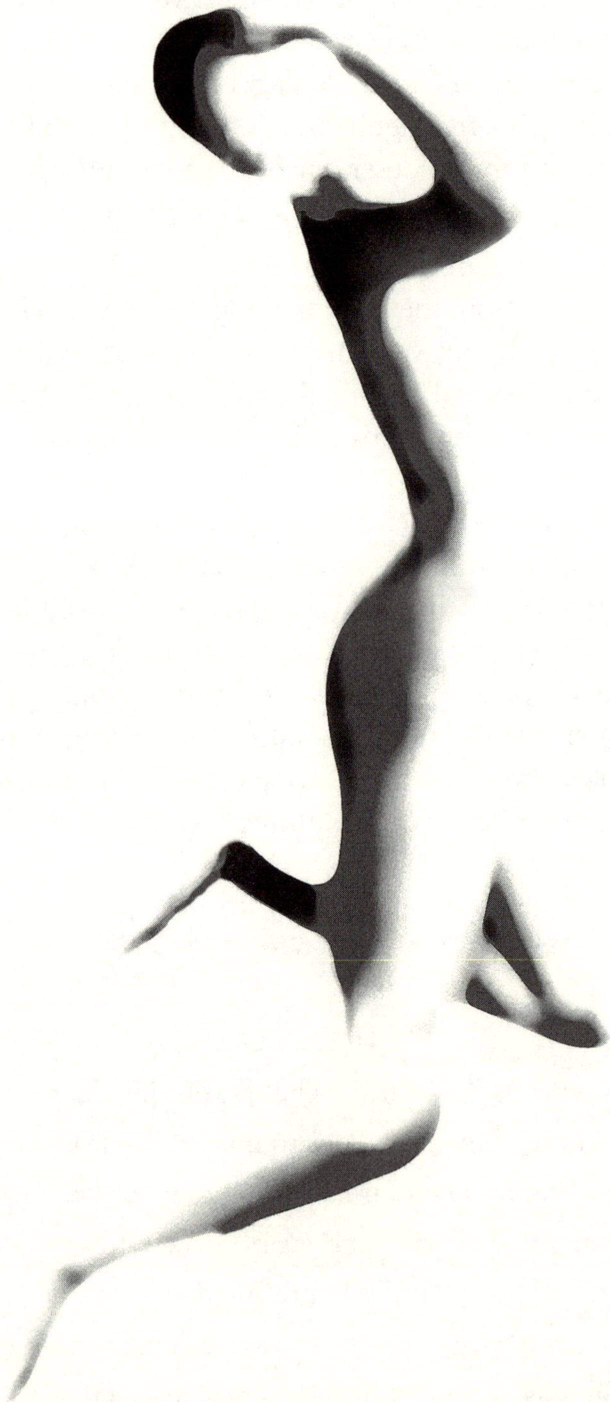

Section Two

NOURISHING NUTRITION

Chapter Twelve

DIETING, NUTRITION, FATS, AND EVERYTHING ELSE YOU WANT TO KNOW ABOUT FOOD

You are about to embark on an incredible journey, one where you will find new information that will challenge some of what you have been taught in the past. Don't worry; I won't try to turn you into a granola-eating, tree-hugging extremist. The bases of the *BetterBody BetterLife* program are common sense and real-life execution. I created the plan from years of fine-tuning my own life and from the feedback of people I coach. I created the plan with you in mind.

Think about food and nutrition with a logical mind-set and without the influence of the decades of media and governmental propaganda that we all have experienced. We are often influenced without our awareness. Food products are seamlessly incorporated into sitcoms, cartoons, and movies to influence our purchasing decisions. Athletes endorse a product because they are paid megadollars, not because they believe in the product. Industries force and lobbyists buy the government's endorsement or assistance — indirectly of course.

At the risk of sounding like a conspiracist, I'll ask you to consider the funding sources for "expert unbiased" studies. The original food group pyramid that most of us grew up with is now retired. Its development was funded mostly by animal-agriculture industries and related trade councils. It does not take a genius to see the connection. Is it then a coincidence that the National School Lunch Act stipulates that meals include meat, or a meat alternative such as cheese or dairy products? We all remember how disgusting school lunches taste, but did you know that, according to the USDA, school lunches are higher in sodium, saturated fat, and fat than recommended for a healthful diet? Maybe the slogan should be, "No fat children left behind." It's no wonder most Americans are confused about health and nutrition.

Of course, some things were the best advice possible for their time; not everything is a form of corruption. Many things that we once believed are no longer considered true. The process of studying and observing over the long-term with increasingly more precise tools yields new information. Many products on the market today were not even imagined 40 years ago. My point is, choose carefully. Consider where the information is coming from and ask yourself if it is logical. Does it make sense? What are the benefits? What are the side effects? Is there a better option? The only one who can make the best decision for you…is you! You must be the gatekeeper of your mouth and your mind and decide what will go in both.

Thankfully, things are starting to change for the better. The latest version of the food pyramid is better, but it still has many flaws. Many schools now have better choices, restaurants are offering healthier options, and some supermarkets are specializing in the healthy lifestyle. Even some media are investigating and reporting more truthfully about the food industries. Some savvy reporters are blogging their findings without an editor as a gatekeeper. We are now getting information directly from unbiased sources.

"DIET" IS A FOUR-LETTER WORD

How many times have you tried a diet without success? If your answer is "many times," then you know firsthand that diets are temporary and ineffective. Stop the yo-yo effect. Instead of dieting, learn and use the fundamentals of physiology and nutrition. This section contains the core knowledge you need to become fit, lean, and healthy. You will find no magic potions or remedies here, only the principles on which to build a foundation for your life. Learn the methods for living well, and you will always be on the right path. You will never "diet" again. Please, don't say that word.

To be healthy and fit, you need the *Trilogy of Health* to work in synchronicity. Three elements of nutrition, cardiovascular conditioning, and muscle toning must be tended and performed regularly. They must work in harmony. I am not emphasizing the importance of one over the other. However, nutrition is essential to living well. Without proper nutrition, the human body cannot function at its full capacity, nor will it have the energy to perform the physical components of a healthy and active life. Remember, the *BetterBody BetterLife* plan requires less than 3 percent of your day. You can follow it without using premade foods or ever setting foot in a gym.

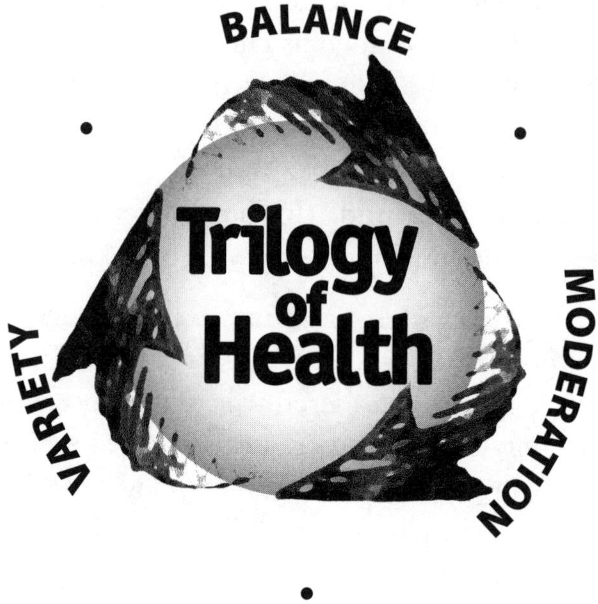

THE BETTERBODY BETTERLIFE TRILOGY IN HEALTH PHILOSOPHY
PROPER BALANCE, VARIETY, AND MODERATION

I've found that most people know little about proper nutrition, and many have a lot of misinformation. These deficiencies explain, in part, why nearly two-thirds of Americans are overweight. We think that we know how to eat properly, but the truth is that most of us have only a vague idea. Most of us did not learn about food through formal education. We learned our food habits from our parents. Unfortunately, our families may have taught us to take huge portions, employ high-fat cooking methods, and relish high-calorie desserts. Fad diet books, advertisements, the news, and conversations with friends also contribute to our misinformation about nutrition. As a society, we have deviated far from the basics of human physiology. Trends lean toward chemicals, pills, fad diets, and miracle elixirs — the quick fixes. We are inundated with advertisements that guarantee results with no effort or exercise. We are bombarded with claims of "the cure" with no scientific or testing research on products that are not regulated by the government. We are told to believe that our doctors can prescribe a pill that will lower cholesterol without significant side effects. If you expect to find a miracle elixir that will let you shed weight without effort, you will be unhealthy for the rest of your life while you wait and try every "new" product under the sun.

By changing your habits, you can change your life. You can dramatically increase your life expectancy and your quality of life. The lower risk of certain diseases in other cultures can be attributed to dietary and lifestyle differences. The reverse is also true. Only in America does a person order a double burger with mayo-sauce and cheese, large fries, a large soda — and then jumbo-size it! To add to this atrocity, the meal is then inhaled on the run. Countries that are currently experiencing an invasion of fast-food restaurants are experiencing cultural and physical changes. These countries now have climbing obesity rates that were previously low and stable.

TIME FOR CHANGE

You must make changes if you want to evolve from a state of obesity to the splendor of fit living. If you do not eat properly and sensibly, you cannot lose weight and live healthily. Perhaps you don't want to give up the foods that you enjoy. You don't have to. You can still have many of the foods you love, but in moderation. In other words, eating a slice of pizza or a chili-cheese dog on a regular basis is not advantageous to fitness management. However, having one on occasion is acceptable and reasonable. I know people who are overweight and want to lose weight, but they won't change their eating habits. Many people are simply resistant to change. An overweight person who continues to make the same choices will continue to be overweight. Period! It's the definition of insanity. Those same people will continue to complain about a spare tire, difficulty moving, lack of energy, back problems, loss of strength, how old they look, and how old they feel. They will be talking about losing weight until the day they die, and that day will be sooner than it has to be — much sooner. What are you going to do? Talk about losing weight for the rest of your life or start controlling your weight and life today?

NOT A DIET

Of course, you like the foods that you eat currently, but you are conditioned to them. Just as people from India are conditioned to spicy food and the Japanese are conditioned to eat a lot of seafood, many Americans are conditioned to eat processed fast food. Living a life on processed food may be commonplace in the U.S., but it is not normal for the human body. What may seem like change and sacrifice at first will become normal over time. You will enjoy new favorites. Healthy eating requires your body — or more specifically your mind — to learn the new menu choices. Soon your taste buds will adapt and dictate new favorites. You will discover that the foods of healthy living are enjoyable and fun to eat. Best of all, you won't feel any guilt. Healthy foods do not have to be "rabbit food," and you don't have to eat like a health-food fanatic. Healthy meals are not bland, boring, or repetitive; they can be exciting, fun, and delicious.

Do not say "diet" when referring to your eating behavior. When I use the word diet in the *BetterBody BetterLife* plan, I am referring only to the food that you consume, not "being on a diet." The *BetterBody BetterLife* philosophy is a logical, holistic (holistic means dealing with the body as a whole), sensible, and effective method to permanent weight loss so you live a fit and healthy life. Your body has dietary needs, and the food you consume is part of your daily diet, or dietary intake, but you will never diet again. In the first chapter, we talked about how the contemporary term [to] "diet" is a gimmick designed for rapid, short-term weight loss, typically through highly selective, restrictive, and ridiculous regimens. "Diets" are often unhealthy, unproductive, and even unsafe. Sure, you can lose weight with many "diets," but they are not a permanent solution to the lifelong struggle that we all face. "Diets" do not address realistic long-term plans for living. Stop struggling and start living

WEIGHT LOSS IS EASY

Calories are a measure of the energy content of food. The mechanics of weight loss can be summed up in a simple mathematical formula:

WEIGHT LOSS FORMULA	
+ CALORIES IN - CALORIES OUT - CALORIES USED = WEIGHT GAIN OR LOSS	• If you eat more calories than you use for energy or excrete as waste, you gain weight. • If you eat fewer calories than you use for energy or excrete as waste, you lose weight. • If the amount is about the same, you remain at a steady weight.

This formula is why diets work, but they do not keep weight off. If you restrict your calories on any diet, you lose weight. However, you quickly gain the weight back when you return to your old habits. As you have probably experienced, weight loss is possible, but keeping weight off is another story. Living fit keeps this mathematical principle in balance for a life without dieting.

THE EATING PLAN

The body is like a machine. It needs fuel for energy. The body operates most efficiently when it has small amounts of fuel (food) throughout the day. When a person consumes more food than the body can process or eliminate, the excess gets stored as body fat. If the body is fed appropriate amounts of fuel (food) throughout the day, it can process the energy efficiently and no excess is stored as body fat. Fueling your body five times a day is ideal, but such frequent eating can be unrealistic given our hectic schedules. So, what can we do?

Eat three meals a day plus two midmeals (formally known as snacks) in between. Snacks have a negative connotation because they are often sugary and fatty foods, such as donuts, candy, chips, cake, and others. A midmeal is more than a snack; it is a minimeal or a proper, healthful, refueling serving of food. The *BetterBody BetterLife* plan starts your day with a balanced breakfast, or powerfest, as I call it. I use this term because this is the meal that jump-starts your metabolism and powers your day. This meal minimizes cravings throughout the first half of the day and gives you the energy your body needs to function optimally. Next, you will have a midmeal to keep you going and to stave off cravings. Then, you will enjoy a full and balanced lunch to power your afternoon. You will then have another midmeal in the afternoon to keep your engine running until dinner. At dinnertime you will enjoy a balanced meal. You should be finished with your last meal at least 2 hours before you retire for the night. This time gives your body a chance to digest your food before you are horizontal for 8 hours. In the coming chapters you will learn in detail how and what you need to do for each meal. Ready?

TIRED OF BEING TIRED?

In my twenties, I was the poster boy for bad dietary habits. I often hear from clients that they, too, are poster children before they start my program. They consume chili-cheese dogs, double burgers, cheese fries, a big piece of chocolate cake, and a jug of soda–and that is just for lunch! Greasy foods and sweets are a part of daily

MEAL PLAN EXAMPLE

6:15	A.M.	Wake up
7:00	A.M.	Powerfest
9:30	A.M.	Morning midmeal
12:30	P.M.	Lunch
3:00	P.M.	Afternoon midmeal
6:30	P.M.	Dinner
10:00	P.M.	Sleep

life–often every meal. What's worse, they often eat an oversized meal right before going to bed. When I was eating that way, I realized that I was growing a spare tire and that I did not sleep well. I was always thinking, "Why am so tired?" Even though I had acquired an extensive knowledge of healthy nutrition since my teens, I ignored the facts when I was young and thought of myself as immortal. We all come to a point in time when we realize that we're not as indestructible as we would like to think. During my enlightenment, I increased my knowledge through research and learned how to replace bad habits with healthy ones to improve my energy level and sleep.

When I changed my eating habits, my body took a short time to adjust, but once it did, I stopped missing the foods that I had once craved so intently, and my energy level skyrocketed. This will happen for you, also. After a short adjustment period, your body will adapt to new foods and a new eating style. In fact, you will crave healthy foods and find your old habits offensive. You will see people eating the way you used to and wonder, "How did I ever enjoy eating like that?" Now I have lost my uncontrollable desire for the chili-cheese dogs that I once lived on. I promise that the same change will happen for you once you change your eating patterns.

Food dictates many aspects of your life. If you eat well, you will sleep better, have more energy, handle stress better, and look better. Living a life of healthy nutrition and exercise, you will feel great and improve your odds of living to a healthy, ripe old age. Best of all, you will feel more alive, and you will be mentally alert. One of my goals is to go scuba diving on my one-hundredth birthday. Anyone want to join me?

I hope that your eating habits are not as bad as mine were. However, if they are, I can assure you that after your body goes through a brief transformation, you will have no regrets, nor will you go back to the way you were. You don't have to give up your favorites; however, I'm willing to bet that your favorites will change.

WHAT ARE YOU GOING TO DO?

TALK ABOUT LOSING WEIGHT FOR THE REST OF YOUR LIFE OR START MANAGING YOUR HEALTH AND LIFE TODAY?

Chapter Thirteen

FOODS OF CHOICE

This chapter is Nutrition 101. You know that you need to eat foods that are good for you. But what are these foods? They're probably foods that you have been eating your whole life, perhaps on a regular basis. Often we simply overindulge and consume too much food. Even if you are eating the right food, you will still gain body fat if you consume more calories than your body needs or can eliminate, no matter what the food type. Eating too much of a good thing is not a good thing. If you eat only foods that are unhealthy, such as processed foods, the effect is multiplied, and the body gains fat even more rapidly.

In the pages that follow, you will learn about the types of food, their benefits, and the number of servings you should consume each day. You will learn why it is so easy to gain body fat and so hard to lose it. You will learn about the preparation methods that are best for fat loss and the proper quantity for each serving. In this chapter, you'll find strategies and tips to assist you in your journey. Whether you prepare your own meals, buy food on the run, or eat out at a restaurant, you will have the knowledge and the awareness you need to make appropriate choices and achieve your objectives.

This section will challenge some of your food beliefs. Some of the concepts that you have accepted all your life are not true. Some of the information presented in the mainstream media is not true. Some conventional wisdom about food is not true. The *BetterBody BetterLife* plan is based on common sense and holistic knowledge gained from many cultures and from many scientific studies.

PROTEIN

Protein is the most important element in nutrition. The word comes from a Greek word that means "primary" or "first." In quantity, protein is second only to water in the body. The brain, blood, muscles, tissues, and every cell in the body require protein, and the body is composed primarily of protein. Just as it needs oxygen, every cell in the body requires protein for metabolic activity (Metabolic activity or metabolism is the process of building up and breaking down of substances in the body to provide energy and nutrients to sustain life.) Protein allows your muscles to repair and grow, and it gives you long-term energy. Protein is the only food source that contains nitrogen. The body constantly loses nitrogen through urine, stool, skin, hair, and nails; therefore, protein needs to be replenished continually. Nitrogen is a component of the vitamins necessary for good health. Proteins are made of nitrogen-containing subunits called amino acids, which are the building blocks of all the body's proteins. Amino acids are crucial to a healthy body because they build, repair, and maintain body tissues.

The 20 amino acids can be divided into two groups: essential and nonessential. Eight essential amino acids (nine for children) need to be acquired through daily food intake. The human body cannot produce these eight essential amino acids; therefore, it must obtain its supply from food. The body can manufacture 12 nonessential amino acids from the essential amino acids if needed. This sounds technical, and it is. The good news is that you do not need to be a nutritionist to understand proteins and live a healthy lifestyle. Simply put, if you are eating a well-balanced diet of quality foods, you will get plenty of quality protein including all the essential amino acids.

Chicken, fish, and beef are usually the first protein sources that come to mind, but the list is much longer. Poultry, pork, eggs, legumes (beans and peas), nuts, soy (tofu), and dairy products supply protein. Even fruits and vegetables supply some protein. Except for pure fat (oil, butter, margarine) and pure sugar, all foods contain at least some protein. In addition, every food has a different composition of amino acids. Foods that supply all eight essential amino acids in similar proportions to the body's requirements are called high-quality or complete proteins. Proteins from animal sources, dairy products, and soy are considered complete. Vegetables are incomplete protein sources because they lack one or more of the eight essential amino acids. However, plant foods can be combined to supply all eight essential amino acids. For example, rice and beans, natural trail mix, peanut butter on whole-grain bread (jelly fruit spread optional), and tortillas and beans are "complementary" because together they supply all eight essential amino acids. Complementary foods do not have to be eaten in the same meal, or even on the same day, but included regularly in meals.

Most Americans believe that meat should be the main part of the meal and that vegetables are a side dish. Forget that idea. Meat should be a small part of your meals. If you are eating a well-balanced quality diet, a 3 to 4 ounce serving of animal meat protein per day offers more than enough nutrients for a healthful diet. That isn't much if you're accustomed to three quarter-pound hamburgers or 16-ounce New York strip steaks. Eating like Fred Flintstone belongs in the Stone Age. Forget the traditional meal of a huge steak and french fries, which will probably give you indigestion and certainly give you high cholesterol. As a rule of thumb, a serving of steak or chicken breast will fit in the palm of your hand and be of similar thickness. Your hand is your built-in measuring device.

A main health issue with animal products, such as bacon, hamburgers, and chicken skin, is their high fat content. Some animal meats are certainly better than others, but all meat products should be consumed in moderation. To make matters worse, some cooking methods, such as frying, add a large amount of unneeded fat. If you want a surgeon to do a Roto-Rooter job on your arteries before you reach fifty, eat a lot of fried meat. With the proper knowledge, choices, and preparation, you can eat a variety of lower-fat, animal protein foods. For example, when preparing meat, trim all excess fat and remove the skin on poultry. Grill or broil meats so that fat can drip away. If a recipe calls for two eggs in an omelet, eliminate the second egg or both yolks. The yolk contains most of the egg's fat and cholesterol. It is a good idea to limit whole egg consumption to two a week.

If I told you about the processing facilities of meat producers and packagers, you would probably never eat meat again. Even many "free range" animals are brutally slaughtered in horrific, inhumane ways. The animal-

PROTEIN GROUP

(Meats and Beans) 3 servings a day

Food Serving	**Serving sizes equal:**	
Meat, poultry, fish	3-4 ounces, cooked and lean	
Soy burger	5 ounces	
Dried beans, peas or lentils	1 cup	= 2 oz meat
Eggs	1 egg	= 1 oz meat
Tofu (made from soybeans)	1/2 cup tofu	= 1 oz meat
Peanut butter	2 tsp	= 1 oz meat
Nuts	1/3 cup	= 1 oz meat

(Whole eggs are high in cholesterol and fat; they should be consumed in moderation)

Protein Choices

Beans	Black eyed peas, lentils, pinto, and kidney are just a few to choose from.
Beef	Lean cuts with all fat trimmed.
Buffalo	Very lean, healthier than beef, and farm raised.
Chicken	Skin removed before cooking White meat is healthier .
Complementary vegetables	Eat a wide variety of vetables and fruits every day to get the essential amino acids.
Eggs	Limit to two servings a week; limit to egg whites, when possible.
Fish	Salmon, blue, swordfish, and haddock are a few of the better choices.
Meat alternate	Vegetable substitutes such as meatless meatballs and meatless sausages.
Ostrich (Emu)	Low fat – similar taste to beef with lower fat and cholesterol.
Soy	Soy beans, soy milk, and tofu. Choose organic products.
Turkey	Low-fat like chicken.

processing industries paint an idyllic portrait of processing techniques and the benefits of eating meat. Frankly, the system is brutal and disgusting.

I am often asked if I eat animal protein such as meat and fish. I do, but I limit these foods to a few times a week, and I meet my protein needs mostly through plant sources such as vegetables, beans, and soy. Some people call me a vegetarian, but they are wrong. I am a healthy eater; that means I eat mostly organic, plant-based foods, but I do not limit myself to those foods because nearly all foods have health benefits. I thrive on a balance of all healthy foods. Life is about balance.

I choose to limit my intake of meat because the human body has a difficult time digesting meat. Meat consumed in large quantities has a horrific effect on the cardiovascular, respiratory, and endocrine systems, as well as on overall health. A diet rich in meat is a ticking time bomb. I also believe there is a correlation between mass-produced animal meat and cancer because of the way that animals are raised, fed, genetically altered, and injected with growth accelerators. When I eat meat, I buy the freshest and most naturally raised animal meat I can obtain locally. It costs more, but I know it has the least amount of impurities. It is a fundamental investment in my health.

PROTEIN CONCLUSION

Protein is important to health. All cells require it, and it aids in building and repairing the body. Too much or too little jeopardizes health. Protein is found in plant and animal products. The average American consumes more than twice the amount of protein from animal products than is needed for good health. Exercise caution in the types of protein consumed because animal proteins can often be high in fat. Fried chicken, sausage, hamburgers, and other high-fat protein sources promote the storage of extra calories as body fat. Choose protein foods that are low in fat and include an abundance of vegetables in your diet.

"Excessive animal protein is at the core of many chronic diseases."

T. COLIN CAMPBELL, PROFESSOR OF NUTRITIONAL BIOCHEMISTRY, CORNELL UNIVERSITY IN *THE CHINA STUDY*

Chapter Fourteen

CARBOHYDRATES

Fad diets have given carbohydrates a black eye. "Carbs" are blamed for everything from obesity to hyperactivity. It is not carbohydrates that cause weight gain and other health issues, but simply consuming too many calories and too much of the wrong types of food. As an affluent, industrialized nation, we have increased our consumption of processed sugars (sweeteners like corn syrup) dramatically while decreasing our consumption of natural carbohydrates (grains). With industrialization, the people of our nation have grown heavier. This same trend is happening in developing nations around the world.

Carbohydrates are not the culprits. The villain is the overconsumption of simple carbohydrate products processed with fat and sweeteners, such as pastries, white bread, cookies, candy bars, and pasta mixes. Their harmful effects have led to scorn for all carbohydrates. Sensationalism about carbohydrates confuses people and makes understanding proper nutrition more difficult. Some sly entrepreneurs and advertisers use this confusion to sell bogus products, such as "trapping" pills.

The truth is that carbohydrates provide energy in the form of glucose (blood sugar) directly to the brain, central nervous system, and muscle cells. Regardless of the type of carbohydrate, the body breaks it down into the simple form of glucose for use in the body. Although all carbohydrates break down in this same way, different carbohydrates break down at different rates. Some provide a rapid energy boost. Others have a longer breakdown time so they supply energy over a longer period.

In an overfat body that is transforming into a lean and healthy body, carbohydrates help the muscles utilize protein. As the body tones and the muscles become stronger, muscles need protein for growth and repair. A proper diet that includes varied and proper carbohydrates allows the protein to be used by the muscle, while the carbohydrates are used for energy. The body needs high-quality carbohydrates.

Carbohydrates can be confusing, so let's clear things up. Most food contains some carbs. Vegetables, breads, fruits, pastries, soda, and candy all contain carbohydrates. The "good carbs" are natural carbohydrates such as vegetables, grains, beans, and fruit. When choosing bread, choose whole-grain breads and pasta over processed white breads and pasta most often. The more a carbohydrate has been processed, the worse it is for you. Avoid or limit processed and fat-laden carbs such as pastries, candy, white bread, and soda. Refined carbohydrates will only add padding to your hips and waist. Say no to carbs that add little or no nutritional value, such as sugar (sucrose), corn syrup, and fructose. Be aware that many food products contain corn syrup, even salad dressings.

Most people have to be consciously aware of not overconsuming carbohydrates. Carbohydrates can be low in calories and nutrient rich when chosen appropriately, and they help in the digestion of other foods. Quality carbohydrates are essential to a healthy diet; they are your allies in weight loss and a healthy lifestyle.

A serving of carbohydrates is the equivalent to 1/2 - 1 cup of ready-to-eat cereal or 1 slice of bread (read the label). If you start your day with cereal and toast, then have a sandwich for lunch and pasta with dinner, you have consumed five or six carbohydrate servings without even trying. Throw in a bagel (equals two to four servings depending on its size) for the morning midmeal and a couple of dinner rolls at supper, and you've consumed 12 or more servings of carbohydrates in one day. Add in some pastries for dessert and you have way overdone it. It is easy for some people to consume 20 or more servings of refined carbohydrates a day. Are you one of them?

It is easy to eat three or four dinner rolls when you're in a restaurant and waiting for the entrées to be served. A medium-sized dinner roll contains 85 calories and has 2 grams of fat. So that predinner bread can add up to 340 additional calories and 8 grams of added fat. Top each roll with butter, and the fat total can soar to more than 20 grams. At home, a double or triple serving of pasta can add an additional 400 calories and 2 grams of fat for plain pasta; it can add as many as 900 calories and 20 grams of fat for pasta in a sauce mix (instant pasta and sauce mix meals in a bag or box). Watch out for high fat and sugar in premade foods, such as instant cereals, breads, and snacks. You may think you are being good when you have a bran muffin for your midmorning meal, but some of those jumbo muffins from the bakery are actually two or three servings loaded with refined carbs and unhealthy fats!

Carbohydrates can be separated into two categories:

- Simple carbohydrates: monosaccharides, disaccharides
- Complex carbohydrates: polysaccharides; starch and fiber

Simple carbohydrates have only one or two sugar molecules.

Monosaccharides (*mono-* means one and *saccharide* means sugar) are the simplest form of sugar molecules, having only a single sugar unit. They include glucose, which supplies energy to the cells, brain, and central nervous system; fructose (fruit sugar); and galactose (from milk products).

Disaccharides (*di-* means two) are a chemically paired combination of glucose, fructose, or galactose sugar units. Disaccharides in a sugary snack can give a quick boost of energy and a bad crash later.

Examples of Simple Carbs

- Brown, raw, cane sugar
- Corn sweeteners
- Corn syrup
- Fructose (fruit sugar)
- Fruit juice concentrate
- Fruits
- High-fructose corn syrup
- Honey
- Lactose (milk sugar)
- Maple syrup
- Molasses
- Sucrose (table sugar)

Complex carbohydrates, or polysaccharides (*poly*- means many) are structurally more complex, hence the name. Complex carbohydrates are the best quality sources to include in your diet. Great examples are whole grains and green vegetables. Starches and fibers contain chains of sugar units reaching into the hundreds or thousands. Complex carbohydrates take longer to break down, so they provide an extended supply of energy.

Starches come from plant foods that can only be digested after cooking. Starches come encapsulated with an indigestible cellulose coating. Cooking softens the coating and releases the starch particles. After consumption, the body then breaks down the polysaccharides for use as energy over an extended period of time. Many starches are beneficial for body-fat loss, as they are low in calories and relatively high in nutrients. Their bulk also creates a "full" feeling. An example of a beneficial starch is a small baked or boiled potato.

EXAMPLES OF COMPLEX CARBS

- Whole grain breads and cereals
- Starchy vegetables
- Beans (also a good protein source)
- Whole-wheat pasta
- Peas
- Brown rice

Fiber is different because the body cannot digest it, but it is a great promoter of health. Fiber has been called the "body's broom" because it speeds the digestive process, increases regularity, and prevents

FIBER LABELING

Look for breads with whole wheat or whole grains on the ingredients list. The first ingredient is the greatest by quantity and the last ingredient is the least by quantity.

Whole-wheat bread must be made from 100 percent whole-wheat flour. "Wheat bread" may be made partly from refined flour and may have caramel coloring for appearance.

High fiber: 20 percent or more of daily value

Good source of fiber: 10 - 19 percent of daily value

More or added fiber: at least 2.5 g more per serving

More information on nutrition labels: http://www.cfsan.fda.gov/~dms/foodlab.html

constipation. Fiber adds bulk to make meals more filling without adding many calories. Fiber can be found in foods that are nutrient rich and that appeal to everyone's tastes.

Fiber is divided into two categories, soluble and insoluble.

Soluble fibers are sticky, and they gel with water. Soluble fibers can also reduce cholesterol in the blood, and they can help the body regulate its use of sugars. Soluble fibers are abundant in fruits, oat bran, barley, and dried beans and other legumes.

Insoluble fiber gives structure to plant cell walls. Also known as roughage, it passes through the digestive tract with nearly no change in form. Insoluble fiber absorbs large amounts of water. It helps move stool through the colon to prevent constipation. Good sources are wheat bran, whole-grain products, and the skins of fruits and vegetables.

Although the body does not digest fiber, it is important to health and weight management. Those who eat a varied and balanced diet don't need to increase their fiber. However, most of us don't consume enough fiber. Increase your intake by substituting refined (white) flours with whole-grain flour products and eating plenty of fruits and vegetables.

EXAMPLES OF FOODS THAT CONTAIN FIBER		
Grains	Grapefruit*	Spinach*
Oatmeal*	Oranges	Sprouts*
Pasta	Pears	
Popcorn	Prunes*	**Vegetables**
Rye*		**(cooked)**
Wheat pasta*	**Vegetables** (raw)	Asparagus
Whole-grain flour*	Celery *	Carrots*
Whole oats**	Green pepper	Broccoli*
Whole wheat*	Lettuce	Green beans
	Legumes**	Parsnips*
Fruits**	Kidney beans*	Peas**
Apple w/skin**	Lima beans	Potato w/skin*
Apricot	Navy beans*	Spinach*
Banana*	Lentils	Zucchini
Blueberries*	Mushrooms	

*Higher in fiber (within group) – ** High in soluble fiber

The glycemic index rates foods for their effect on blood glucose levels. It is a scale that runs from 1 to 100. The higher the glycemic index rating, the faster a food is absorbed in the body. High-glycemic-index foods cause blood sugar and insulin levels to spike quickly and then crash just as quickly. Such foods include processed white bread, pastries, candy, and bagels. Generally lower glycemic index ratings provide a longer and steadier energy supply. These are foods based on oats, barley, bran, and whole grains, such as oat bran, sweet potatoes, beans, and soy.

GLYCEMIC INDEX EXAMPLES

LOWER GLYCEMIC 55 AND UNDER	MODERATE GLYCEMIC 56 - 69	HIGHER GLYCEMIC 70 AND ABOVE
Most nuts	Banana	White bread
Most beans	Brown rice	Pineapple
Whole grains	Honey	Watermelon
Broccoli	Oatmeal	Popcorn
Low fat yogurt	Ice cream	Potato
Grapefruit	Raisins	Pumpkin
Yam / Sweet potato	White rice	Corn flakes
Carrots	Sugar	Bakery foods
Oranges	Pizza	Syrup

With all of these variables and different opinions, how can you be anything other than confused? Some diets add to the confusion by not allowing potatoes and corn. Some even argue no peas or broccoli. Such restrictions are ridiculous. Every natural food has a place in your diet. If you make your dietary plan difficult and restrictive, you will go crazy, fail to follow the plan, and gain even more weight. Keep it simple. Choose "nature's foods" — vegetables, fruits, and grains most often. Limit processed white breads, processed junk food, and sweets. This advice sounds like common sense, doesn't it? If you are going to eat something that converts to blood sugar quickly, balance it with lower glycemic foods to minimize the glucose fluctuations. So go ahead and enjoy corn-on-the-cob when you barbecue.

Note: If you are diabetic, the glycemic index is very important. You need to monitor your carbohydrate consumption closely. Consult your physician for guidance.

That was probably more about carbohydrates and fiber than you wanted to know.

Here's a summary:

- Choose natural carbohydrates over processed ones.
  Examples: Vegetables, fruits, and whole-grain breads, cereals, and pasta
- Simple carbohydrates: Avoid or limit refined carbohydrates.
  Examples: Corn syrup, white bread, pastries, sweet junk food, soda
- Complex carbohydrates: Substitute for simple carbohydrates.
  Examples: Whole grains, wheat, dried beans and other legumes
- Be aware that many products have added sugars. Check food labels.
  Examples: Corn syrup, sucrose, fructose, glucose, lactose, dextrose

Easy ways to include complex carbohydrates and fiber in your diet:

- Choose quality "nature" foods such as vegetables, fruits and grains.
- Use the reminder "5 – 4 – 3 a day."
  Five vegetables, four fruits, and three grain servings a day.
  Leave the skin on fruits and vegetables when possible.
- Replace refined white grains with whole-grain or whole-wheat products.
- Pasta cooked al dente (firm) is better because of a lower glycemic response.
- Add fiber to your breakfast.
  Examples: fiber-rich cereal, oatmeal, whole-wheat waffles, or whole-bran products.
- Include legumes in your meals several times a week (beans, peas, or lentils).

CAUTION: Avoid fiber enhancers, such as pills and fiber supplements. High doses of fiber can wreak havoc in the digestive system and cause injury. Ouch!

EXCESS IS BAD. MODERATION IS GOOD!

CARBOHYDRATE CONCLUSION

Although the body breaks down carbohydrates to simple sugars — in the form of glucose, which the body utilizes as energy — eating a diversity of healthy carbohydrates is important. Different kinds of carbohydrates are processed at different rates, giving the body short- and long-term supplies of energy. An assortment of vegetables, grains, fruits, starches, and fiber in the diet is a sure way to get adequate amounts of nutrients and maximum and balanced energy. Your body performs better and feels great when you

CARBOHYDRATES
5 - 4 - 3 a day
5 vegetables, 4 fruits, 3 servings a day of whole grain

One Serving Size Equals:

Bread - Whole grain or wheat is best	1	slice
Bagel (small) or English muffin	1/2	
Uncooked ready-to-eat cereal	1	cup
Cooked cereal	1/2	cup
Rice (dozens to choose besides white)	1/2	cup cooked
Pasta (try whole wheat pasta too)	1/2	cup cooked
Couscous (type of pasta)	1/3	cup cooked
Tortilla	1	
Fat-free pretzels	1/2	cup
Wheat crackers (low-fat)	4	crackers
Popcorn (w/o butter or salt)	3	cups popped

give it an ample supply of quality foods. As in your car, bad fuel in the system will cause it to sputter and gasp or simply not run at all. Feed your body with high-quality energy sources to keep it running like a finely tuned sports car.

"The first wealth is health."

RALPH WALDO EMERSON

Chapter Fifteen

NUTRIENT RICH

FRUITS AND VEGETABLES

Nature's convenience foods — often portable and portion-sized — fruits and vegetables are a key source of nutrients that you can enjoy throughout your day. It's easy to take an apple, banana, orange, grapes, celery, carrots, and dozens of others with you wherever you go. All such foods are excellent sources of an array of vitamins, minerals, antioxidants (counteracts the damaging effects of oxidation), fiber, carbohydrates, and protein that the body requires for optimal health.

A body that consistently lacks enough nutrients will perform poorly, and it can develop diseases and chronic health issues. "[Thirty] percent to 40 percent of all cancers are directly linked to the foods we eat, the exercise we get, and how well we watch our weight, " says the American Institute for Cancer Research (www.aicr.org) in *Food, Nutrition and the Prevention of Cancer: A Global Perspective.* Consuming an assortment of fruits and vegetables is required for a complete and balanced lifestyle. Instead of processed snacks, fill your shopping cart with choices from the produce department.

There are many ways to consume enough fruits and vegetables each day, even if you are traveling or spending a lot of time at work. Vegetable leftovers from dinner can make a great nutritional addition to lunch, or they can become a great midmeal. Plus, taking leftovers from home for lunch at the office saves money. You can also add fruits and vegetables to salad and pasta.

> **Caution:** Vegetables often come with high-calorie toppings (such as sour cream or cheese sauce), and fruit may come prepared with added sugars (for example, canned fruit in syrup). Beware of the product you are consuming and avoid options that contain many needless calories.

VEGETABLE GROUP

This one is a no-brainer. You probably know that you should eat more veggies. Did you know that vegetables should be in every meal? If you want more energy, eat more veggies! Make vegetables the foundation of your meals, not a side dish. Forget the old concept of meat as the main event on your plate; get green nutrients on center stage. They are called green nutrients because they are nutrient rich, low calorie, and (often) green. Actually, great vegetable foods come in a wide array of colors. Make no mistake; all vegetables are wise choices that benefit your health. Many vegetables can be considered "free" foods. They are cholesterol free, low in fat, low in calories, and rich in nutrients. You are free to eat a lot of vegetables. Most meals fall short on nutrients, and many professionals neglect to emphasize green nutrients in their "diet plans." If you are hungry, eat extra vegetables first, instead of meat, pasta, bread, or other foods high in fat and calories.

POTATOES

Potatoes are not the villains they are made out to be. At about 100 calories for a medium-sized baked potato, a potato is a low-calorie food. Potatoes are also fat free, cholesterol free, high in vitamin C and potassium, and rich in vitamin B6 and dietary fiber. When prepared properly, they can be an excellent choice in your diet. Be careful about the toppings and preparation style you choose, as they can add hundreds of calories to an otherwise healthful meal. A baked, white potato has a high glycemic index; however, a baked sweet potato has a low glycemic index. If choosing a potato, choose sweet potato or yams most often. Try making baked (instead of fried) potato sticks from potatoes, yams, or sweet potatoes.

LOOK AT THESE EXAMPLES; THEY ARE YOUR WEIGHT LOSS FRIENDS

All are less than 40 calories per serving. (Excludes sauces and toppings)
Note * = 20 Calories or less per serving

Artichokes	Kale*
Asparagus*	Leeks*
Bamboo shoots*	Legumes (beans - kidney, lentil, lima, navy) †
Beans (Snap, green, yellow)*	Lettuce (choose leafy)*
Bean Sprouts*	Mushrooms*
Beets (boiled)	Mustard greens*
Bok choy*	Mixed vegetables
Broccoli	Okra
Brussels sprouts*	Onion
Cabbage*	Peas (Chinese)
Carrot (and juice)	Peppers*
Cauliflower*	Pumpkin
Celery*	Radicchio*
Chicory*	Radish
Collards*	Sauerkraut*
Collard greens	Spinach
Corn on cob	Squash*
Cucumber*	Tomato*
Eggplant	Turnips*
Endive*	Turnip greens*
Escarole*	Vegetable juice*
Green pepper	Watercress*
Green beans*	Zucchini*

† Although beans are higher in calories than the choices above, they are an excellent low-calorie choice, and qualify as a good source of protein.

GIVE GREEN NUTRIENTS A THIRD

Nutrient-rich vegetables should fill one-third of your plate. That amount will allow you to fulfill your nutrient requirements while adding quantity to your plate, but with fewer calories. This strategy ensures that you eat enough food to feel satisfied, yet minimize the number of calories you consume. It also ensures that you get a high-quality balance of nutrients in your diet.

Get five vegetables servings or more per day. A meal can easily have two servings of vegetables. For example, you can indulge in one-half cup each of mashed sweet potatoes and broccoli florets, or you can start with a spinach salad and then have some asparagus with the meal's main course. A glass of vegetable juice is a serving of vegetables. For spalike refreshment, add a few cucumber slices to a glass of water and eat the cucumber. As with any food, caution in preparation is the key. Avoid using high-fat cooking methods.

VEGETABLE GROUP **5 servings a day**	
Serving sizes equal:	
Cooked vegetables	1/2 cup
Raw vegetables (non-leafy)	1/2 cup
Leafy vegetables	1 cup (lettuces)
Potato (baking, sweet or yam)	1 small (3 ounces)
Vegetable juice	3/4 cup (6 ounces)

FRUIT GROUP

This group gives you a boost of antioxidants to help ward off the free radicals (highly reactive chemicals that attack molecules) that cause some cancers, heart disease, and many other disorders. With the physical stress our bodies have to endure, you will benefit from the protection and rejuvenation that fruit has to offer.

Fruits, with the exception of avocados, are very low in calories. The calories in most fruits are almost exclusively from carbohydrates, or fruit sugar. That does not make them carbohydrate bombs. In fact, many fruits are moderate to low on the glycemic index. Fruit is low in calories and rich in nutrients, vitamins, and minerals. Therefore, it does not present the carbohydrate issue that some diet plans want you to believe. The nutrients you get from an assortment of fruits in your diet are invaluable for your health. Reach for a banana, orange, or another fruit instead of chips or a candy bar. Enjoy four servings of fruit a day.

Avocado note: Most people mistake this fruit for a vegetable. Avocados are high in calories from fat. However, it is good fat, which is beneficial to health in moderation. Avocados are a healthy part of a balanced lifestyle. Make some guacamole and enjoy it as a part of a healthy meal.

Fruit is an easy and fun food to include in your day. Start off with a cup of orange juice, add a banana or pear during the day as a snack, and have fruit as a dessert. Few people realize that fruit can add zest to a main course. Tangerine chicken, pineapple spinach salad, and mango coconut salmon are just a few ways to enjoy fruit as an entrée. Frozen fruit can be an easy way to get additional servings a day. Add frozen fruit to a dessert or make a fruit smoothie. Fruits are great sources of vitamins A and C and of the mineral potassium.

FRUIT GROUP 4 servings a day	
Serving sizes equal:	
Berries	1/2 cup
Chopped, cooked, or canned	1/2 cup (4 ounces)
Dried fruit	1/4 cup (not too much)
Fruit juice	3/4 cup (6 ounces)
Grapefruit, papaya or mango	1/2 fruit
Whole fruit	1 small

Gimmick Warning: Many store-bought fruit cups contain sugar syrup, which adds unwanted and unworthy extra calories. Choose fruit cups prepared and stored in water; better yet, make your own from fresh fruit.

If the label does not say "pure juice," or "100 percent fruit juice," the product is likely a sugar-filled drink with flavoring. The sugar-filled drinks aimed at children offer no health benefits, so be sure to read the label. They are very sweet with added sugars (corn syrup) and contain very little, if any, real fruit juice.

FRUITY IDEAS

- Grab fruit instead of a candy bar.
- Add flare to a salad. Add orange slices, dried fruit, or raisins.
- For breakfast or dessert, make a fresh fruit juice smoothie.
- Sauté fruit with your dinner to add flare to a main dish.
- Make smoothie Popsicles for you and the kids.
- Keep dried fruit for snacks. (Avoid those with added corn syrup.)
- Have fresh fruit and sorbet for dessert.
- Mix orange and mango juice with seltzer water.

VEGETABLE AND FRUIT CONCLUSION

The bottom line is that most people do not eat enough servings of fruits or vegetables. Include vegetables in every meal, filling one-third of your plate. Eat at least five servings of vegetables a day. Include four or more fruit servings in your daily diet. Choose natural products over processed foods. If it didn't come directly from Mother Earth, think twice about its value.

"The way you think, the way you behave, the way you eat, can influence your life by thirty to fifty years."

DEEPAK CHOPRA

Chapter Sixteen

THE MILK SHOP

Are you ready to have your food beliefs challenged again? Dairy products such as milk are not the panacea that many want you to believe. Dairy products are not the staple that we all grew up on. In fact, you should limit dairy products in your diet. According to nationally recognized author of many nutrition books Suzanne Havala Hobbs, dairy is not needed for health.

Milk products are a good source of calcium and riboflavin. Milk, cheese, yogurt, cottage cheese, and buttermilk are all part of this group. Getting enough calcium is important for bone health. However, there is no correlation between a diet rich in dairy products and better bone heath. A diet high in dairy products may increase the risk of some heart conditions and some cancers (such as prostate and ovarian).

The milk industry's "Got milk?" campaign is a brilliant, multimillion-dollar marketing plan designed to make American consumers believe that they need a lot of milk to be healthy. Athletes and movie stars promote dairy products in the same way that celebrities promote fast foods. Why does milk, the purported great source of bone strength, need to be promoted? The advertising supports the dairy industry, not our health. Dozens of Congressional leaders receive millions of dollars in campaign funding from the dairy industry or its affiliates. In addition, the dairy industry partially funds public school nutrition planning. It doesn't take a genius to see the conflict of interest.

Animals never drink the milk of other animals. Humans and their domestic companion pets are the only animals that drink milk beyond childhood or drink the milk of another animal. In an animal's natural habitat, consumption of milk ends when it's weaned from the mother's breast. Humans stop drinking breast milk as toddlers. So, why do human adults drink from the cow's breast?

DAIRY GROUP Limit to 2 servings a day Serving sizes equal:	
Cottage cheese	1 cups
Evaporated milk	1/2 cup
Frozen yogurt	1 cup
Ice cream	1 1/2 cups
Milk or buttermilk	1 cup
Natural cheese (cheddar, mozzarella, swiss)	1 1/2 ounces
Low-fat Processed cheese (American)	2 ounces
Ricotta cheese	1/2 cup
Yogurt	1 cup

Another concern is that cows are pumped full of hormones, antibiotics, additives, and high-protein supplements to force milk production from a natural production of 16 pounds per day to 50 pounds per day. Animals are also selectively bred and genetically manipulated for increased milk production. Pumping animals full of hormones, antibiotics, and protein supplements and then drinking their milk is not logical. How would you feel if your boss pumped you full of chemicals to get you to produce four times the amount of work each day?

> "The [USDA's] recommendation to drink three glasses of low-fat milk or eat three servings of other dairy products per day to prevent osteoporosis is another step in the wrong direction."
> - Harvard School of Public Health

Am I telling you not to eat dairy products? No, but I am suggesting that you consume them with prudence and choose organic products whenever possible. Dairy is an easy way to get certain nutrients that we need, so it can be included in your dietary plan. Choose dairy products that are low in fat. Whole, 2 percent, 1 percent, and no-fat (skim) milk have very similar nutritional values, but you get fewer calories and less fat from the low-fat or no-fat choices. Reduced-fat and low-fat cheeses are just as tasty as the full-fat varieties. Limit your dairy products to two servings a day.

Need calcium? Green leafy vegetables are a good source. Fortified orange juice and multivitamins are also good sources. Need vitamin D? Regularly enjoy the sun for 15 minutes.

SOME SOURCES OF CALCIUM

- Dark green leafy vegetables
- Fortified orange juice
- Fortified soy milk
- Milk
- Cheese
- Buttermilk
- Cottage cheese (good protein source)

Warning: Butter, cream, cream cheese, and sour cream are not considered dairy products. They are made from the cream that naturally separates from unhomogenized milk. These foods contribute only minute amounts of nutrients to the body; they are very high in fat. Use very sparingly.

DAIRY CONCLUSION

Moderation is the key. This nutritional group can be high in fat, and it has come under a lot of scrutiny recently. The health benefits are debatable and controversial. You need nutrients such as calcium from dairy products or green leafy vegetables and vitamin D from dairy products or the sun. Choose dairy products that are lower in fat and limit your portions to two servings a day. Organic dairy products are the best choice.

"Failure is success if we learn from it."

MALCOLM FORBES

Chapter Seventeen

FRIED OR DIPPED IN CHOCOLATE?

This category should be the smallest part of your daily food consumption. The body requires some healthy fat for the function of the brain and for the transport of vital nutrients. However, you don't need to be concerned about getting enough of this food group. Be concerned about getting too much. Most Americans consume a staggering amount of sweets and fats in their diets.

Sweets and fats are brutally bad for health. Certain foods are triple whammies! When sweets and fats take the place of better nutritional choices, you get a triple whammy of bad fats, high calories, and low nutritional benefit, which virtually guarantees weight gain and obesity. Multiply those whammies by a sedentary lifestyle and you have the epidemic we are experiencing in the U.S. right now.

Fats are loaded with calories. Carbohydrates and proteins have 4 calories per gram. Fats have 9. Furthermore, fats are more readily stored as body fat. Obviously, you should limit or eliminate sweets and fats from your diet. Don't add any fat to meals, because you get more than enough fat from cooking and from your protein sources such as meat. Fat is often "hidden" in other foods. In "Fat Facts," you will learn more about good fats and bad fats.

TIP! When recipes call for a high-fat ingredient, try substituting a low-fat ingredient. For example, use skim milk instead of whole milk or use applesauce instead of oil in baking. Use the Internet to search for ingredient substitutes. Although all fats have 9 calories per gram, unsaturated fats (good fat) are a better choice than saturated fats if fat must be used in a recipe. Use caution when purchasing prepared meals and convenience foods because they are often high in fat. Candy bars and the like have a tiny place in a healthy diet. Have one occasionally, but pass up this kind of snack most of the time.

Fats and sweets can be part of your diet, but they should be incorporated with caution and in moderation. Yes, you can have a dessert dipped in chocolate or fried food specialty when you go out to dinner at your favorite restaurant. Keep in mind, however, that too much indulging will pack on the body fat. Often you can make choices that are more satisfying but contain less fat and fewer calories.

FOODS TO AVOID

Limit all fats and sweets as much as possible.

Bacon	Ice cream
Butter	Jams and jellies
Cakes	Margarine
Candies	Meat fats
Cocoa butter	Palm kernel oil
Coconut oil	Pastries
Cookies	Processed meats
Cream	Salad dressings
Donuts	Sausage
French fries	Soft drinks
Fried chicken	Sour cream

Buyer beware! "Fat-free" products are not the magic elixir that you may have dreamed of. Sweet products (often desserts) that say fat-free on the label may be free from fats, butters, and oils, but they may add a surprise to your waistline. The product may be technically accurate in its labeling, but it is likely a high-calorie product. Treats of this kind are often high in calories because extra sugar is added for taste, and extra sugar means extra calories! Excess calories convert to body fat. Many of these products are good choices compared to their full-fat counterparts, but use caution when purchasing them and read the labels. Fat-free products may not mean "body-fat-free" for you.

SWEET AND FAT CONCLUSION

Avoid sweets and fats most of the time. High-calorie foods such as candy bars, pastries, and desserts will pack on the body weight at an alarming rate when consumed regularly. You can have it fried or dipped in chocolate, but in moderation. You need some fat in your diet. In "Fat Facts," you will learn more about good fats and bad fats.

"If you do not change direction,
you may end up where you are heading."

LAO TZU

DAILY NUTRITIONAL SUMMARY

- 5 Vegetables: 5 or more servings a day
- 4 Fruit: 4 or more servings a day
- 3 Grain: 3 servings a day
  Choose whole-grain options most often.
  Bread, rice, and pasta carbohydrates
- Milk and dairy (Limit to 2 servings a day)
- Protein
  Meat – 1 serving a day (chicken, turkey, fish, beef)
  Choose beans, nuts, seeds, and soy most often.
- Sweets and fats. Avoid or limit as much as possible.
  Choose unsaturated fats most often.

Chapter Eighteen

THE H_20 FACTOR

You know that the body needs water to survive, but do you know why? The simple answer is that all the chemical reactions that keep you alive occur in water. Water is the essential component of your cells, tissues, and organs. Studies have shown that over 50 percent of American adults are chronically dehydrated. This deficiency is not immediately life threatening, but it is a factor in weight gain. Chronic dehydration does not allow the body to perform its normal functions optimally, and it can reduce your life span. Consuming at least five glasses of water a day reduces the risk of heart attacks and stroke by as much as 50 percent according to *The Adventist Health Study*. Like a plant, we flourish with ample amounts of water each day. At birth, water is about 80 percent of your body weight but only 50 percent in the elderly. Are you like the wilted, but living, plant, or are you like the well-watered, flourishing plant?

How long can a person survive without water? .... A few days

How long can a person survive without food? .... More than a month

WATER'S FUNCTIONS

Virtually all of the body's functions require water: digesting food, absorbing nutrients, transporting materials, building tissue, and maintaining temperature. Water is in the cells, the spaces between the cells, and in the blood plasma. It is used to carry nutrients to cells and to excrete wastes from the kidneys, gastrointestinal tract, lungs, and skin. Water is also used in the brain, spine, and joints, and it helps protect organs.

The water excreted through breathing and perspiration serves as part of the body's climate control system. When the body overheats, sensors in the skin send a message to the brain to stimulate the sweat glands to release perspiration. This release cools the body's core temperature. In addition, the body excretes about 1 quart of sweat daily without exertion or noticeable perspiration. Throughout the day, the body releases undetectable amounts of perspiration and undetectable water vapor during breathing.

Water accounts for about three-fourths of muscle tissue, but only about one-fourth of body fat. Therefore, a lean person's body has a higher percentage of water than an obese person's. An obese person who is on a diet that causes water loss, such as a high-protein diet, may face an increased risk of heat exhaustion symptoms, such as weakness, headache, dizziness, and a weak, rapid pulse, because the diet reduces water . This risk can be critically dangerous for obese elderly people. Always supply your body with a generous amount of water.

HOW MUCH WATER?

As little as 1 percent loss of water starts dehydration. The body's primary gauge for water need is thirst, which is a fail-safe indicator. If you wait until your body signals you to hydrate (drink fluids), too much time has already passed since you last hydrated your body. If you consume only enough water to quench your thirst, you will not drink enough to compensate for daily losses or to keep the body performing optimally. Too little water is often a problem in children if they are not taught to hydrate often, and it's a serious concern for seniors.

The body loses 2.5 to 3 quarts or more of water in an average day. That means that you need to consume about 10 to 12 cups of water a day. If you are saying, "I will float away if I drink that much water," you may be relieved to learn that only 8 cups of pure water are needed daily when a person has a balanced diet. That is only four typical size (16-ounce) bottles of water a day. The difference comes from the water in foods. Fruits are of 85 to 90 percent water; meats, 45 to 65 percent; and bread, 30 to 35 percent.

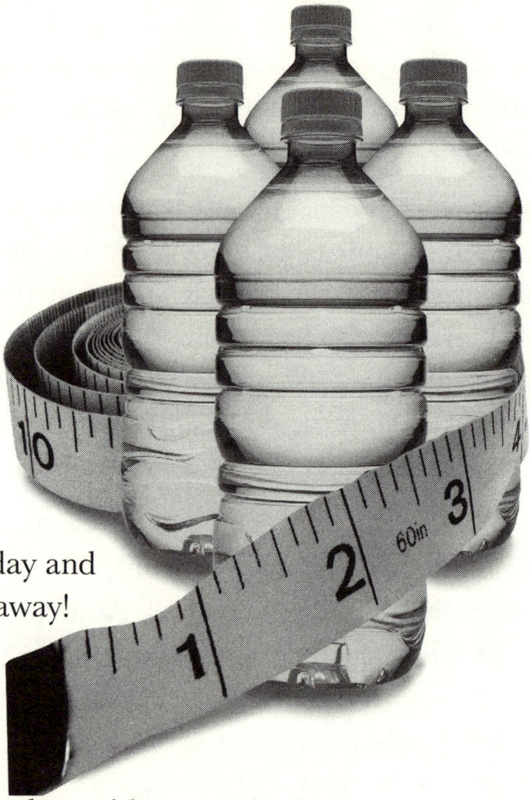

Drink 4 bottles a day and keep the doctor away!

TIP! On hot days or on days with extra physical exercise, consume additional water to compensate for greater water loss.

The first and last thing that you should do for your body each day is drink a cup of pure water. In the morning, your body has gone without water for 6 to 10 hours during the night, and the body loses and uses water 24 hours a day. Therefore, it is best to replenish the body's water as soon as possible when you rise. Drink a cup of pure water with each meal and each midmeal. Add some pizzazz to your water by dropping in a slice of lime, lemon, or other fruit. You can even enjoy the pleasures of a spa by adding cucumber slices to a glass of ice water; then close your eyes and imagine the tranquility of a Calistoga mineral bath.

Not drinking enough water may cause you to feel hungry. Water is a slight appetite suppressant. You may think your body is calling for food, when in truth you are dehydrated. It may not be food that you need, but water. To help ward off those midday munchies, keep yourself well hydrated.

SOFT DRINKS

Soft drinks (soda or pop) account for most of the fluid intake in the diets of many Americans. They are not a great source of water. Although soda contains water, the caffeine it contains is a diuretic, which causes the body to excrete water. What's more, drinking three cans of soda each day can add 450 calories to the diet. A single large cola from a fast-food restaurant (32 ounces) is more than 300 calories.

When consuming a soft drink, you must account for the calories it contains and also for the possibility that it will take the place of a more nutritious selection. If these considerations are taken into account, then soft drinks can be consumed in moderation. A 12-ounce can of soda contains between 140 and 180 calories from approximately 9 to 12 teaspoons of sugar (in the form of high fructose sugar). Soft drinks contribute to carbohydrate (sugar) overload. Diet soft drinks contain saccharin, or aspartame, instead of sugar. Although these products provide few or no calories, be cautious because of the chemical additives diet drinks contain.

FRUIT DRINKS

Fruit *juices* are 100 percent fruit juice. Fruit *drinks* are nothing more than water, high fructose syrup (sugar), and juice flavor or a minuscule amount of added fruit juice. Fruit drinks are high-calorie, sweet-tasting products aimed at kids. Avoid them because they offer little or no nutritional benefit. Many times fruit drinks are worse than soda. Choose fruit *juice* products that contain 100 percent real fruit juice. Genuine, 100 percent fruit juice contains all sorts of vitamins, minerals, and antioxidants. Different juices contain different mixtures of these highly desirable nutrients. Fruit juices contain sugars which mean calories. Those calories need to be factored in to your diet.

COFFEE AND TEA

Have you ever wondered why Americans are so high strung? It could be from the caffeine in coffee. Although coffee-related health issues are debated passionately, no serious adverse effects arise from consuming caffeine in moderation. Excessive amounts, however, can overstimulate the heart, dilate the arteries, and trigger irregularities in heartbeat in susceptible individuals. Caffeine is also a diuretic, meaning it causes excess urine excretion, which in turn promotes dehydration. Consume an extra glass of water for every cup of coffee consumed to compensate for the diuretic effect. In excessive amounts, caffeine can reduce vitamin absorption and cause vitamin deficiencies because of its diuretic action.

Excess is bad. Moderation is good!

Caffeine is absorbed from the digestive tract into the tissues and organs in as little as 5 minutes, and it reaches its peak in about 20 minutes. Caffeine stimulates the central nervous system. In some people, caffeine suppresses fatigue and increases alertness. In excessive amounts (as little as 1 cup of coffee for some people), caffeine can create insomnia, nervousness, irritability, and restlessness. Tea also contains caffeine, but in lesser amounts. Many herbal teas are naturally caffeine-free and therefore a better choice than coffee.

ALCOHOL

Alcohol is a depressant, a sedative, and a diuretic. It has been called the antinutrient because it can interfere with the absorption of nutrients into the body. It offers no nutritional value, but it adds calories and kills brain cells.

One or two alcoholic drinks can add 300 to 900 calories. Since all alcoholic drinks contain approximately the same quantity of alcohol (ethanol), the difference in calories comes from added sugars or creams. Three drinks a day can add as much as 50 pounds of body fat a year. This is not an effective approach to fitness management. Just because you drink light beer, don't assume that your beverage has fewer calories. Some are simply lighter in color.

	Wine	Shot	Beer	Wine Cooler	Mixed Drinks
Calories	**110**	**100**	**150**	**150 – 300**	**150 – 300**

One serving contains:
1 oz shot, 5-ounce wine, 12-ounce beer, 12-ounce wine cooler, standard sized mixed drinks.

In moderation, alcohol can be a part of your diet. (Consult your physician.) Many medical professionals believe that a glass of red wine a day is beneficial to health. However, recent studies question that assertion. In any event, all physicians agree that alcohol consumed in excess causes brain, liver, kidney, cardiovascular, and gastrointestinal damage and sometimes death. Alcohol can cause sexual dysfunction, birth defects, and mental disorders. It can also make you fat.

DRINK RESPONSIBLY. NEVER DRINK AND DRIVE.
AVOID EXCESS - MODERATION IS KEY.

A FLUID CONCLUSION

Water is needed for digesting food, building tissue, transporting nutrients, and disposing of toxins. Water helps protect organs; it is the fluid portion of blood plasma. We have all heard that we should drink a lot of water, and now you know why. I used to hate to drink water. I thought it was tasteless and boring, but when I stopped eating excess soda, sugar, and a lot of other garbage, my taste buds became keen and alert and water began to taste good. Water replenishes and cleanses the body. Let water be a part of your day. Drink four bottles daily.

"Well-being is attained by little and little,
and nevertheless is no little thing itself."

CITIUM ZENO

Chapter Nineteen

FAT FACTS

Do you know that you need fat in your diet? Some fats are good, but how can you know how much dietary fat is good or safe in a diet? With some popular "diet" plans touting high-fat, high-protein regimens, and others recommending low-fat or no-fat, it is hard to tell. After you read the next few pages, you will understand how and why the body can accumulate fat so easily and why it can be so hard to lose body fat without a comprehensive program. In the next chapter, we will examine the common diets of today — and why they won't work. We'll also reveal what the diet plans do not want you to know.

Some dietary fat is required for good health. Dietary fat transports and stores vital nutrients. The human body needs a small percentage of body fat for survival. Fat is responsible for the regulation of temperature and the production and regulation of hormones. It also cushions vital organs. However, the typical American diet is much too high in bad fats. The American Heart Association, the American Cancer Society, the National Cancer Institute, the American Dietetic Association, and most physicians recommend reducing fat intake and decreasing body-fat levels for those who are of an unhealthy weight and body-fat percentage. Yes, there are people who, because of medical issues, have more difficulty regulating body fat, but glandular and medical problems account for much less than 1 percent of the overweight and obese population.

JUST THE FAT FACTS

The human body is dreadfully efficient at storing body fat. We evolved into fat-storage machines as a means of survival. In the era of early humans before we discovered farming, we were hunters and gatherers. Sometimes food was scarce and the quantity was unpredictable, so a reserve of body fat might well spell the difference between survival and death.

In recent history, humans have mastered farming and raising livestock to the point where a consistent and plentiful supply of food is no longer an issue, at least not in the developed world. In the last century, transportation has improved so much that we can now easily obtain nearly any type of food or food product grown or processed anywhere in the world. Technology is maximizing every aspect of the food industry and life. You can now order anything on the Internet without talking to a single person. Everything from automobiles to cooked meals can be delivered to the front door while you are still in a bathrobe sitting on the couch.

These may be phenomenal conveniences, but our waistlines suffer. In the last century, the weight of the average American has increased dramatically. In the era of technology, we are getting larger and larger, in part because more jobs are done from behind a desk and the level of physical activity required for work has continually declined. We don't even have to get up off the couch to change the 450 channels on the tube. Seventy-eight percent of American adults are sedentary. Think about it. Early in the last century, Henry Ford was still developing the car, the first air flight had just taken place, and about one-third of the American workforce was employed on a farm. Few processed foods were available. People had to walk, ride a horse, or raise plants and animals for their own food.

Today, even active adults are packing on pounds from high-fat, high-calorie processed foods. Food is abundant. We overindulgence. We consume in excess. Now our modern bodies store fat simply because they cannot burn or eliminate all the excess. In a world of processed foods, calories add up at a dizzying rate.

If you consume more calories than your body can use or eliminate, the body has no choice but to store the excess energy as body fat. That last sentence is so important that I will repeat it. When you consume more calories than your body can use or eliminate, the body stores the excess as body fat. Most body cells, with the exception of adipose (fat) cells, can only store a limited amount of body fat. Adipose cells store most excess fat. The fat cells in an obese person are thought to be 50 to 100 times larger than those of a healthy-weight person. The number of fat cells can also increase in adulthood to accommodate additional fat. Although the number of fat cells cannot be reduced, fat cells shrink when excess fat is used for energy and body fat is reduced.

When more calories (energy) are consumed than are required for muscular, metabolic, and digestive activities (muscle toning, cardio conditioning, and nutrition respectively), the excess is stored as fat.

Conversely, when more calories (energy) are required than consumed, fat cells break down stored triglycerides and release fatty acids into the blood. Cells that are in need of energy can then break down those fatty acids. These lipid fragments are then combined with a glucose fragment to burn as energy. That process is the reason why very-low-carbohydrate diets are neither safe nor effective. Carbohydrates supply the glucose fragments required to supply energy when the body is calorie deficient.

Blah, blah, blah! What does this mean? It is all technical mumbo-jumbo. Who cares, Croix? Tell us how to lose weight. Okay, simply put: Eat natural healthy foods most often and burn more calories than you eat and you will lose body fat. You must combine proper nutrition with cardiovascular exercise and muscle toning.

It is really as simple as that. The most important part of body-fat loss is consistency and your "why." Why are you trying to lose body fat? You must have a strong enough "why" or you will not follow through.

WEIGHT LOSS FORMULA	WEIGHT GAIN FORMULA
+ EAT HEALTHY	+ EAT JUNK FOOD
+ EXERCISE MORE	+ EAT TOO MUCH
+ TONE MUSCLES	+ BE SEDENTARY
= WEIGHT LOSS	= WEIGHT GAIN

AS WE AGE

We are almost doomed to gain weight as we age if we do not adapt to the body's metamorphosis. As you grow older, you need fewer calories. The caloric needs of an average man or woman of average height and weight decrease by about 15 percent over 30 years. This might sound like a small amount, but if a woman continues to eat like a 20-year-old without an increase in activity, she could gain as much as 100 pounds by age 50. For men, the weight gain could be even more. Most often, people are unaware of this fact, and they continue to eat as they did in their twenties. In addition, most adults become less active as they age. If a person is not active throughout life — and most adults are not — muscle mass decreases, which in turn increases the percentage of body fat. That means that a person will get fatter, even if his or her weight remains constant. This, in turn, lowers resting metabolism. Muscle tissue burns calories even when the body is at rest. Less muscle means a reduction in calorie burning and an increase in fat storage.

FAT STORAGE

The human body stores excess dietary fat as body fat. When you consume meals high in unhealthy fat, your body adds body fat more easily and quickly than if you ate meals lower in fat, even if the number of calories is equal. In other words, if you eat a lot of high-fat foods such as candy, potato chips, and ice cream, you will easily gain body fat. If you eat mostly natural, low fat foods, you are much less likely to gain body fat. Food choices make a significant difference.

	Men	Women
Age 20	2,900 Calories daily	2,100 Calories daily
Age 50	2,400 Calories daily	1,800 Calories daily

The chart above represents average healthy, active persons.

During digestion, the human body uses energy (calories) to convert food into fuel. This process is known as thermogenesis. The body burns a portion of food's calories while processing digested food and converting it into fuel the body can utilize. During thermogenesis, the body burns as little as 3 percent of dietary fat in the conversion to fuel. In comparison, the body burns up to 25 percent to convert lean protein or carbohydrates into fuel. This difference is the obvious advantage derived from minimizing fat consumption when losing or maintaining weight and body fat. A person who consumes low-fat, balanced meals burns more calories, in part due to thermogenesis. Dietary fat contains 9 calories per gram — more than double the calorie content of lean protein or carbohydrates at 4 calories per gram. Dietary fat is calorie dense and your body cannot burn it as easily.

1 gram of fat	= 9 calories
1 gram of protein	= 4 calories
1 gram of carbs	= 4 calories

Fats are a necessary part of every person's diet. You cannot survive without them. Dietary fats are required in small amounts and are responsible for a variety of functions. Fat-soluble vitamins such as A, D, E, and K cannot be fully absorbed into the body without fats to dissolve and transport them. Fats, to some extent, also make some foods more pleasurable.

FAT LABELING

Fat Free Less than 0.5 grams of fat per serving

Low Fat 3 grams or less of fat per serving

Reduced Fat At least 25% less fat per serving as compared to traditional food

Less Fat Same as reduced fat

Light Meal "Low fat" – at least 50% less fat per serving; "low calorie" – at least 1/3 or fewer calories per serving

Low-fat Meal 3 grams or less fat per 100 grams, and 30% or less from fat

Saturated Fat Free Less than 0.5 grams saturated fat and less than 0.5 grams trans-fatty acids per serving

Low Saturated Fat 1 gram or less of saturated fat per serving and no more than 15% of calories from saturated fat

Reduced or Less Saturated Fat At least 25% less fat than traditional food

Calorie Free Less than 5 calories per serving

Low Calorie 40 calories or less per serving

Reduced or Fewer Calories At least 25 percent fewer calories per serving than the nonreduced version

Make sure to read the Nutrition Facts Label to find out how many calories and fat grams are in a food. Pay attention to the serving size listed on the label. The label may state a serving size smaller than the amount you were planning to eat!

FIVE CATEGORIES OF FATTY ACIDS

GOOD

Monounsaturated fatty acids – Liquid at room temperature.

Lower LDL (bad) and raise HDL (good) cholesterol
Olive oils - 72% monounsaturated
Canola - 62% monounsaturated
Found naturally in avocados, nuts, and seeds

Polyunsaturated fatty acids – Liquid or soft at room temperature

Lower LDL (bad) and raise HDL (good) cholesterol
Safflower oil - 78% polyunsaturated
Sunflower oil - 66% polyunsaturated
Corn oil - 59% polyunsaturated
Soybean oil – 44 - 61% polyunsaturated

Omega-3 fatty acids – Fatty acids that are highly polyunsaturated

Found in seafood, such as salmon, tuna, and mackerel.

BAD

Saturated fatty acids – Raise cholesterol

Coconut oil - 87% saturated fat
Palm kernel oil - 81% saturated fat
Butter - 62% saturated fat
Found in animal foods, such as meat, poultry skin, whole milk, and seafood

REALLY BAD

Trans-fatty acids – Fatty acids not found in nature

Raise LDL (bad) cholesterol and lower HDL (good) cholesterol
Formed during hydrogenation, the manufacturing process that makes products more stable at room temperature. Hydrogenation increases hydrogen saturation and extends shelf life.
Examples are margarine, most lard, and vegetable shortening

Not all fats are created equal. Essential fatty acids (the most commonly known is linoleic acid) need to be obtained from foods because the body cannot produce them. Essential fatty acids are necessary for many chemical activities, including proper growth in children, the production of sex hormones, the control of smooth muscle contraction, and the synthesis of cell membranes. Essential fatty acids also prevent dry skin and flaking, and they help regulate heart rate, blood pressure, immune response, and the breakdown of saturated fats. Many scientists also believe that some essential fatty acids may prevent some cancers and lower the risk of heart disease.

Even though unsaturated oils (fats) do not raise blood cholesterol levels, they are calorie dense and will promote the storage of body fat when consumed in excess. Keep this in mind when choosing foods and measuring portion sizes. Fat is abundant in most American diets and must be limited to achieve weight loss and maintain a fit and healthy body. Processed foods generally contain a lot of fat and bad fats. Trim the visible fat from meats. Remove the skin from chicken and trim the white fat from beef. Choose lean cuts of meat that have little marbling. Most foods contain at least some fat, visible or not. Limit or eliminate from your diet high-fat and processed foods such as bacon, sausage, salami, and bologna; solid fats such as lard, butter, and margarine; and snacks or desserts that are high in both fat and calories.

BUTTER VERSUS MARGARINE

This choice between butter and margarine is hotly debated, or at least the advertisers would make you think so. Most diets are too high in both. Both butter and margarine should be limited in the diet. Use margarine sparingly because of its processing and ingredients. Avoid those margarines that contain trans-fats. According to the *Nurses' Health Study*, 4 teaspoons of margarine a day can increase a woman's chance for heart attack by 50 percent.

Use cooking alternatives such as olive oil or applesauce whenever possible. With the proper substitutions in recipes, there is little difference in taste, and often the lighter recipe tastes better. When you must, choose butter over margarine. Butter is a better choice because it is more natural. However, butter is an unhealthy fat and should be limited.

A FAT BOTTOM LINE

Reduce and replace dietary fat intake.

Replace bad fatty acids with good fatty acids.

Replace saturated fatty acids and trans-fatty acids with unsaturated fatty acids.

Use olive oil most often and get a variety of natural fatty acids from foods such as nuts, soy, seeds, and avocados. Replacing saturated fatty acids with unsaturated fatty acids lowers bad cholesterol and raises good cholesterol. Monounsaturated and polyunsaturated fats, the good fats, help prevent many diseases and cancers.

Unsaturated fats = Good
Saturated fats = Bad
Trans-fats = Really Bad

AN EFFICIENT BODY

In health management, whether it is for weight loss or maintaining fitness, you will achieve your goals far more easily with an efficiently operating body. Using the *Trilogy of Health* philosophy, the body becomes an efficient machine. Your resting metabolic rate increases, making your body more proficient at shedding fat.

To be successful at any endeavor, you must have enough information and knowledge. I don't want to overload you with information, but you need enough to make educated decisions. I have assembled the information you need, and I have kept it as simple as possible. As you learn and apply the *BetterBody BetterLife* program, refer back to this information to refresh and reinforce the new knowledge. Repetition is often the best way to learn. Change your habits and you will change your life.

LOSE FAT, NOT WEIGHT

You don't need to lose weight. No, this isn't a typo. You do not want to lose weight; you want to lose body fat. Body fat is the excess storage of fat (in adipose cells) that results from the overconsumption of calories, and it poses many health risks. People do not become overweight; they become overfat, and excess body fat needs to be eliminated to attain a fit and healthy body. If you simply try to reduce your weight, you will lose water, lean muscle mass, and nutrients. That is what happens with most diets — and certainly if you crash diet. You need to lose body fat — not water, not muscle, and certainly not nutrients. You may need to reduce your weight to a healthy level, but you need to achieve that goal by losing excess body fat while maintaining or increasing muscle tone. Without integrating cardiovascular exercise and muscle toning with a healthful dietary plan, you will simply reduce the number on the scale. You will not be leaner and more toned, you will not raise your metabolism, and your body will not efficiently maintain itself. Losing weight alone may not make you healthier. You need proper nutrition, cardiovascular conditioning, and muscle toning to become lean, fit, and healthy.

"You should examine yourself daily.

If you find faults, you should correct them.

When you find none, you should try even harder."

XI ZHI

Chapter Twenty

DIETING DILEMMAS

You have already heard me say that diets do not work. In the last chapter, you learned why fat is readily stored in the body and which types of dietary fats are good and bad. Now you will learn how the two are related and why. In some cultures, overweight is considered a sign of health, prosperity, or fertility; in other cultures, anorexic models are considered icons of beauty. The truth is that neither overweight nor underweight is healthy because both conditions stress organs, create medical complications, and reduce fertility. To be fit and well, you need a healthy body weight (low body fat percentage). A person who is too thin or too fat is neither healthy nor fit.

We are bombarded with pitches for weight-loss gimmicks and fads everyday. Ads about the newest machine, pill, or diet that will make you thin with no effort are everywhere. It is no wonder that we are confused and flustered about what to do. Now we see a new wave of "experts" called certified nutritionists and certified trainers. Often these people have no more education than a 6-hour course with a near-zero failure rate among the students. Many graduates of 1-day courses do not know their gluteus maximus from their elbow.

NOTE: The government is finally cautioning consumers about products that promise weight loss without effort. Be cautious also about products that promise weight loss of more than 2 pounds per week. Fat loss takes time.

What should consumers do? Back to the basics. As Albert Einstein once said, "Things should be made as simple as possible, but not any simpler." Before you continue learning the right things to do, you need to understand why the latest "diets" do not work.

WHY DIETS FAIL

Being "on a diet" is rarely successful because most diets impose unrealistic expectations. Many diets unrealistically limit food choices. While these diets may make good advertising claims and interesting news clips, they almost always fail because they are too restrictive. People who have tried a high-protein diet know it is difficult to go out to a restaurant because half of a typical meal is carbohydrates. Vegetarians also have a hard time because most of a typical restaurant menu are meat dishes. If your meal choices are too restricted, staying on a diet is nearly impossible.

Most diets are an all-or-nothing deal. They are not about constant improvement and a healthy way of living. Most diets are about a radical and unnatural change in behavior that is unrealistic and often unsafe. Some diets cause rapid weight loss, which isn't necessarily a good idea. Never eating again will cause rapid weight loss, too, but it's certainly not a good idea either.

PROTEIN DIETS

High-protein diets are the latest rage. They go by many names, but they all follow a similar formula. They severely limit the consumption of carbohydrates. Advocates of protein diets claim that a body deprived of carbs will burn excess body fat, and weight loss will follow. Some of these plans allow unlimited portions of any type of meat, fish, eggs, and cheese. A high-protein diet does not permit most carbs such as bread, pasta, or potatoes. Weight loss is often substantial in the early period, but the lost weight is water, not fat. Weight loss will then ensue if (and only if) the person consumes fewer calories than the body needs. However, the weight loss includes muscle and water, not fat alone.

The way to a healthy weight and life is through the loss of body fat. Consuming fewer calories than the body uses for metabolic, digestive, and muscular activities causes weight loss, not simply consuming fewer carbs.

The main source of energy for the brain and the central nervous system (CNS) is glucose. Glucose is most easily obtained from carbohydrates, then protein, and lastly from fat. If carbs are not available, then the body degrades proteins to obtain the needed energy source. The body's last resort is to degrade fat into a glucose substitute, its least efficient energy source. The body attempts to supply its glucose from dietary intake. If carbs are unavailable in the diet, the body will utilize lean tissues, such as organs and muscle, for energy. If insufficient sources of carbs continue, the body builds up ketones, the glucose substitute. Ketones cannot serve all the needs of the brain or the CNS, therefore putting health in jeopardy. A person who eliminates carbs from the diet will enter a condition called ketosis, a toxic state caused by a buildup of too many ketones. If the body is completely deprived of carbs for several weeks, death can ensue. In the late 1970s, when the original rage for no-carbohydrate diets began, some deaths were reported when dieters' bodies ran out of a glucose supply, causing the body to "eat" the heart muscle for energy.

The initial weight loss from a high-protein diet is water, because the kidneys attempt to eliminate ketones and the by-products that result from the breakdown of excess protein. When a protein diet is discontinued and carbs are reintroduced, many dieters balloon back to their previous weight or higher. The rebound is not because of the carbs but because of the regain of water weight, the continuing excess consumption of fatty protein foods, and the resumption of carbs from the prediet days. Consequently, the former dieter unwittingly consumes more calories than ever before, causing massive weight gains.

The strongest argument against this type of "diet" is that the excessive amounts of fat from animal protein can increase cholesterol and the risk of cardiac failure. This is not the only issue, just a blatantly obvious one. A protein-only diet also promotes nutrient deficiencies and stresses the kidneys and other organs. This can be a real issue for people with diabetes or liver or kidney problems, as well as for pregnant women.

Diets are designed to be temporary. They limit the variety of foods, often the favorites of most who attempt the weight loss. When limiting vegetables, fruit, and grains on a high-protein diet, you also limit nutrients and antioxidants that are crucial to life. Without a variety of foods, your chances of long-term success are small.

Possible side effects: vitamin and mineral deficiency, headaches, dizziness, fatigue, nausea, constipation, and bad breath. Long-term effects can include organ damage, heart damage, and muscle loss.

FASTING

Fasting fails to promote weight loss because the body goes into a "self-preservation" mode and reduces the number of calories (energy) it burns. When the body is deprived of energy sources, it "anticipates" a shortage in the future and slows the metabolic rate to conserve energy. Repeated fasting causes the body to build up a resistance, making weight loss even more difficult after each successive fasting session.

Fasting, or starving yourself for immediate weight loss, can have even more severe side effects than high-protein diets. Whether you totally eliminate meals or totally eliminate carbs, the results can be the same. These types of diets are often used when the dress for Saturday night's special event will not fit. Although the consequences of short-term use of these methods are not severe, fasting stresses the kidneys and liver each time it is employed. Therefore, fasting is not recommended, nor is it effective in the long run. Limiting meals, eliminating certain food groups, or using very-low-calorie diets will cause some weight loss; however, the loss is mainly water and muscle. Fasting does not result in the desired effect, which is the loss of body fat.

Possible side effects: vitamin and mineral deficiency, headaches, dizziness, fatigue, nausea, liver and kidney damage, and bad breath. Long-term effects can be organ damage, heart damage, muscle loss, and in severe cases, death.

VEGETARIAN DIETS

There are many variations of vegetarian lifestyles. Many people choose not to consume animal foods for health reasons or because of their moral or ethical philosophies. Many vegetarians do not eat meat but consume certain animal products such as milk or eggs. Others eat no animal products at all. Without care and precise compensation to acquire the needed amino acids from acceptable protein sources or complementary sources, a vegetarian diet can cause the body to become deficient in some critical nutrients. The brain, blood, muscles, tissues, and all cells in the body require protein for metabolic activity. That said, a vegetarian lifestyle is an excellent way to live, and possibly the healthiest lifestyle if managed properly. However, a restrictive and improper vegetarian diet will cause significant health issues.

Possible side effects: vitamin, mineral, and various nutrient deficiencies. Poor development of the fetus and inadequate milk production; liver and kidney damage; loss of muscle mass; headaches, dizziness, fatigue, and nausea. External signs of a shortage of protein are dry skin and hair, weak nails, and a frail overall appearance.

LIQUID DIET MEALS

Popularized by celebrities, these diets were all the rage in the late 1980s. In the 1990s, sales plummeted as the same celebrities who promoted the products couldn't keep the weight off. Now liquid diet meals are enjoying a resurgence in popularity due to the potential for rapid weight loss. But fast weight loss means fast regains and then some. Another issue is the quantity of nutrients supplied. Some liquid meals do not provide the proper amounts of nutrients or calories. If meal replacement shakes are the only food consumed, the effects can be severe. Each meal replacement shake is different, and each contains a different mix of nutrients. There is no consistency between manufacturers, and there are few regulations.

Conversely, some shakes, especially those protein shakes aimed at athletes and bodybuilders, can provide ten to 1,000 times more of some nutrients than the body needs. This sort of nutrient overconsumption can have a toxic effect on the body. The body may build up toxic levels of nutrients, leading to organ malfunction with prolonged use. If you want to gamble, go to Las Vegas.

Possible side effects: muscle loss, lower metabolism, heart problems, nutrient toxicity, nutrient deficiency, constipation, hair loss, dry skin, gallstones, and bad breath.

HIGH-FIBER DIETS

Twenty to 30 grams of fiber a day is ideal, but is more a good thing? You decide. Excessive fiber in the diet can cause constipation and dehydration. Bulk fillers (which are high in fiber) reduce hunger by absorbing fluids and then swelling inside the stomach. This can cause obstructions in the intestinal tract, sometimes even requiring surgery to be relieved. Ouch! Need I say more?

Excess is bad. Moderation is good!

THE LAST WORD ON DIETING

Any diet plan that minimizes or eliminates intake of any type of nutrient will cause havoc with prolonged use. And switching from diet to diet is even worse. Whether it's high-protein, low-carb, grapefruit, corn flakes, or cabbage soup, that fad diet will not be effective in the end, and it may cause severe side effects. Many studies show that when prediet habits are reintroduced, the dieter nearly always returns to the prediet weight and usually gains additional weight. The result is a higher body-fat percentage and a higher weight. Diets often cause vitamin, mineral, and various nutrient deficiencies that can create organ, muscular, and neurological disorders and complications. Without appropriate dietary consumption, the body does not have all the components it needs for an effective, disease-fighting immune system. Each nutrient has a specific job and without each nutrient, the body cannot carry out each function required to stay optimally healthy. Falling prey to the hype of the media and advertisers will only keep you fighting the battle of the bulge over and over again.

"Every failure is a step to success."

WILLIAM WHEWELL

Chapter Twenty-One

NEW MEAL HABITS

You can secure a healthy future with healthy habits. Change your habits and you will change your life. *BetterBody BetterLife* is a lifestyle, not a diet or temporary plan. It is a matter of replacing each bad habit with a good habit. It is said that habits cannot be eliminated, only replaced with another behavior that becomes a habit after 21 days. I think it takes longer than that to develop a new habit, especially if you are changing a habit that you have developed over decades. The longer an action is reinforced, the stronger the habit becomes. To develop a healthy, fit lifestyle may take longer because it is a series of habits that need to be replaced and new ones internalized. The important part is that you become aware of your unproductive habits (many of them are unconscious) and that you make an effort to replace them with productive habits that will last the rest of your life.

You probably eat as you were raised. If you are with a partner, your traditions may have fused with your mate's, and you eat with the unhealthy habits of both childhoods. Add these to the bad habits you developed using modern amenities, such as convenience foods, takeout, fast foods, and fad diets, and you have little chance of maintaining a healthy weight.

In this chapter, you will learn how to replace bad habits with good habits. You will learn how to avoid situations that encourage you to cheat and how to use strategies that will help you to succeed. You will not need too long to become accustomed to new routines, but you will need some diligence to reinforce new routines until they become natural and instinctive.

WHAT'S ON YOUR PLATE?

Portion control and balanced meals are big issues in the Western world. Most of us were raised to believe that a big juicy steak should be the main part of the meal, with a heaping pile of potatoes and a small portion of green vegetables on the side. And then your mother told you to eat more. The human body cannot effectively utilize such large, fatty meals. They contain too much for the body to process at one time, and the excess calories cannot be utilized. As you know by now, excess calories are converted to fat. For the body to be efficient, it must take in an appropriate amount of food periodically throughout the day.

Portion control principle: Moderation, Balance, and Variety

In general, portion sizes in the American diet are double, sometimes triple, or even quadruple what they should be. Many of us fill our plates until there is no more space left to fill and then go back for seconds. Overconsumption is why $8.95 all-you-can-eat buffets are so popular. Too many of us eat rapidly until we feel bloated. By that time, we have consumed at least twice what the body needs. The habit of overeating makes the maintenance or loss of weight impossible. Twenty minutes must pass before the stomach sends signals to the brain to acknowledge food consumption. That delay allows people who eat fast to consume too much before their brains say, "Enough." A health-conscious person eats slowly and pauses between bites by putting down the fork, chewing, and then swallowing each bite before eating more. Try that sequence and see how much less you eat. To slow it down even more, have a sip of water between bites. These behaviors will slow down your "plate-to-mouth" speed, and the water will help you feel full more rapidly, so you consume less food and fewer calories. Water also helps digestion. Start a meal with a broth-based soup or a light appetizer; then rest for 10 minutes before starting the main course. You may find that you are nearly satiated at that point and you will need little additional food to have a satisfying meal. Give your body time to adjust and say, "Hey, I like this. Thank you." Your body will begin to expect small meals. Listen to your body and stop eating out of habit.

DON'T COUNT CALORIES

Don't count calories. Count portion sizes. The palm of your hand is a built-in measuring device sized to fit the body it is attached too. The size of the serving should be equal to the surface area and the thickness of the palm (excluding fingers). An average size would be approximately 4 inches square by 1 inch thick. Have a fist-sized portion of starchy foods such as yams, potatoes, and squash. If the serving is bigger than your palm or fist, it is too big. This is an ideal way of proportioning food, because a smaller person has a smaller hand and a larger person has a larger hand. In this way, every person can have a meal that is sized appropriately for his or her body.

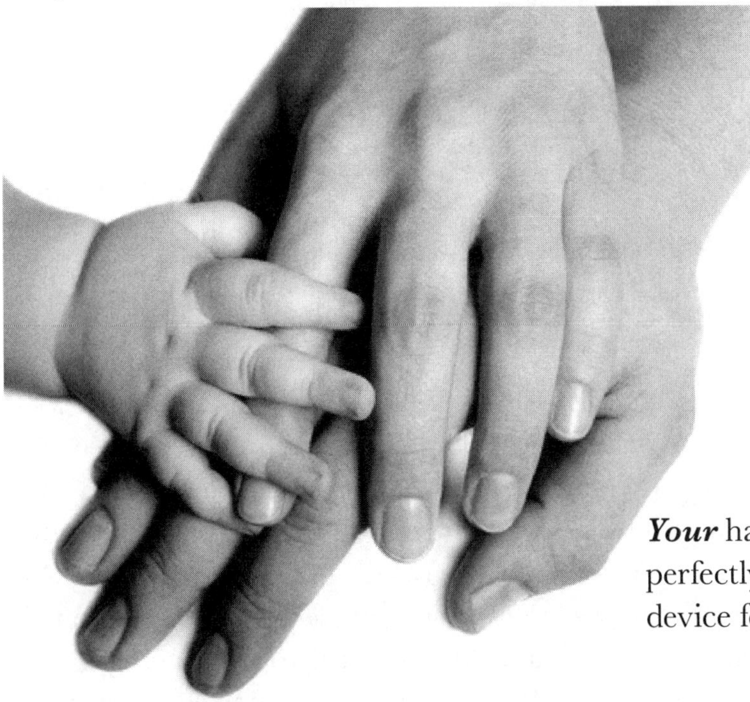

Your hand is a built in and perfectly sized measuring device for your body.

Your plate should be divided into three, similar-sized portions of vegetables (usually green nutrient sources), protein (typically lean meat), and carbohydrates (typically wheat and grains or fruit). Each third of your plate is a palm-sized portion of each food type. As a result, you should serve yourself a palm-sized portion of protein, a palm-sized portion of carbohydrates, and a palm-sized portion of green nutrients. As a point of reference, these three will fill an 8-inch appetizer plate comfortably. The food fills most of the plate, but it does not fall off the edges or have to be heaped on. To be successful at body-fat loss and weight management, the foods on that plate need to be lean, low in fat, low in calories, quality foods, in appropriately sized portions.

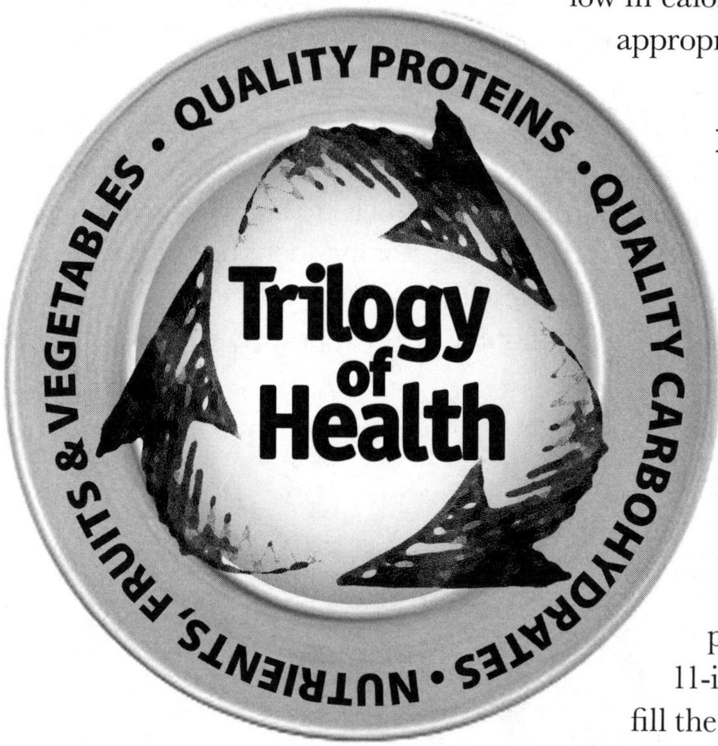

Eat Quality, Not Quantity.

A healthy serving size of lean meat is 3 to 4 ounces; a serving of carbs is typically 1 cup cooked; a serving of veggies typically equals 1/2 cup. Most people eat on a 10- or 11-inch dinner plate and fill the plate with food until the plate disappears. Sound familiar? This is too much food for everyone except a burley lumberjack or linebacker, and even those guys could probably cut back. If you can't resist filling the plate completely, use an 8-inch appetizer plate instead of a dinner plate to force yourself to limit the amount of food you take. Even if you're still hungry after eating that food, wait 10 or 15 minutes before considering seconds. Before you fill your plate again, ask yourself if you need more or if you are merely conditioned to having a second serving. If you decide that you need more, green vegetables are your best choice because they are low in calories and fat.

At first such "small servings" may seem like too little, but they are not. They are the right amount — enough, but not too much. They are the amount your body can utilize most efficiently. We have become a society of oversized meal eaters. We eat until we get a bloated feeling. Many people have been unwittingly overeating all their lives. If you combine proper portion sizes with proper eating habits, you will be satisfied without feeling bloated. After a short period of eating smaller portions, your body will adapt, and you will feel satisfied more quickly and easily.

It is also important to eat on a schedule, even if the time to eat comes before you feel hungry. If you wait until you are hungry or until you "have time" to eat, you are more likely to overeat and to choose foods that are not healthy. If you are not hungry at mealtime, have a small meal or small, healthy snack. It is important to nourish your body regularly throughout the day to avoid cravings and to maximize digestion. The body works most efficiently when it is fed a balanced set of meals from the beginning of the day to the end.

Stick to the following plan, and you will live with nutritional optimization.

Every day: 3 balanced meals
2 midmeals

POWERFEST

Do you start your day with a cup of java and a piece of toast? That breakfast will only add to your love handles. Coffee and toast have so little nutritional value that the body believes it is being deprived of nutrients. Coffee is also a diuretic, which encourages the elimination of water and nutrients. This morning meal puts your body into self-preservation mode and lowers your metabolism.

Starting your morning with a powerfest (what most people call breakfast) gives your body the energy it needs to kick off the day right and to shift your metabolism into high gear. A powerfest is your first meal of the day: balanced and complete — to supply the fuel needed for your morning. When you wake up, your body has been without food or water for 8 to 12 hours. It needs to be replenished with quality energy sources to perform in top form.

If you perform your fitness routine first thing in the morning, then a powerfest becomes even more important. When your body burns large amounts of energy, it needs short-term and long-term fuel sources to help it recover. Because you are probably on the go from the moment you wake up, it is critical that you take a few minutes for a proper morning meal. If you skip your morning meal, your body will quickly go into survival mode, and you will burn fewer calories throughout the day.

A powerfest should include a balanced mix of protein, carbohydrates, fruit, or vegetables. Ideally, you consume your powerfest at a relaxed, sit-down meal, but that kind of time allotment is impractical for many people.

Therefore, you must have a plan to ensure that you get a proper meal in the morning. Prepare your powerfest the night before (perhaps set some leftovers aside?) and have your food ready to grab as you run out the door to school or work.

POWERFEST EXAMPLES		
1/2 grapefruit	Glass of O.J.	Leftovers:
Omelet (1 egg)	1/2 wheat bagel	3 oz chicken
Wheat toast (1 slice)	Cereal w/soy milk	Vegetable medley
Vegetable juice	Banana	Grain toast (1 slice)

MIDMEAL TIME

What do you do when it is midmorning, you're hungry, and you have 3 more hours before lunch? This is the time for your midmeal. Instead of a donut or a candy bar, choose a healthful and balanced snack that will recharge you and give you energy for the next few hours. Your midmeals should be much smaller than your meals, but they should have enough nutritional value to keep you satisfied until the next meal and to reduce your urge to snack. Midmeals should be balanced and healthy. They are opportunities to eat more foods from those categories that you may lack, such as fruits, vegetables, or protein. Make midmeals fun and enjoyable.

A piece of fruit is a good example of a midmeal. Other great options are one-half a wheat pita with some hummus, or some leftovers from the previous night. Just because it is morning, you don't have to have a typical morning meal. Have your dinner leftovers for your morning or afternoon midmeal. I often have leftovers for my midmeal, because there is often not enough left over for a full meal. I sometimes have salad greens, pasta, or a few grilled chicken bits. Midmeals of leftovers can easily fit into small plastic containers to take with you to work or school.

MIDMEAL EXAMPLES

- 1/2 grain bagel, orange
- Yogurt cup, grain crackers
- 1 cup of leftovers (e.g. potato/veggie medley)
- Small garden salad
- Small fruit salad
- 1/2 peanut butter & fruit spread sandwich
- Cup of pretzel nuggets and a banana
- Crackers and hummus dip

LUNCH

The second full meal of the day is especially important. Instead of simply grabbing a quick bite, eat a full, balanced meal. Like your powerfest, lunch will stave off the munchies and give you energy for the afternoon lull. Lunch can still be a quick, easy, and portable meal, but it needs to be complete with protein, carbs, and green nutrients. Good examples for when you are on the run are a veggie wrap or turkey sandwich (protein) on wheat bread (good carb), with lettuce and tomato (some vegetable nutrients) and a touch of light mayo. (Mustard is even more healthful.) You can complete your lunch with some additional nutrients, such as a small salad made from spinach or mixed greens (iceberg lettuce is useless), or a piece of fruit.

Some dangers lurk among your lunch choices. An otherwise productive and healthful lunch can easily become laden with calories and fat. When choosing the topping for a sandwich, choose spreads such as mustard, ketchup, lemon, teriyaki, or hummus because of their low-calorie content. If you choose a creamy sauce, opt for a light- or reduced-calorie option and use very little. Stay away from creamy salad dressings. They add hundreds of calories to your meal. Another danger is portion size. A sandwich can be two, three, or four times the size of a healthful serving. Three ounces of turkey is only three regular slices of meat or five thin slices. Many sandwiches have several times that amount. If your deli gives you an inch of meat, eat only half of the sandwich and save the other half for the next day. Also, be concerned when eating on the run. It is easy to unwittingly overeat when you are rushed.

LUNCH EXAMPLES

- Veggie wrap
- Pasta salad with veggies and fruit
- Turkey and veggie wrap
- Salad with grilled chicken
- Salad with grilled seafood
- Hummus and vegetables
- Chicken pita

DINNER

No longer will your dinner be a Stone-Age food gorging at the end of the day. As we discussed, you will fill your dinner plate with three palm-sized portions: one of protein, one of carbohydrates, and one of vegetables. You will probably sleep better when you have your last meal of the day at least 2 hours before you retire. That period gives your body sufficient time to begin the digestive process while you are still active. (Hopefully you are not sacked out on the couch.)

Dinner gives you the fuel and nutrients you need to replenish and rebuild your body while you rest for the next 8 hours. Choose dinner foods carefully. The process of reducing body fat and rebuilding your physique demands that you make high-quality choices to give your body the best opportunity to progress effectively and rapidly.

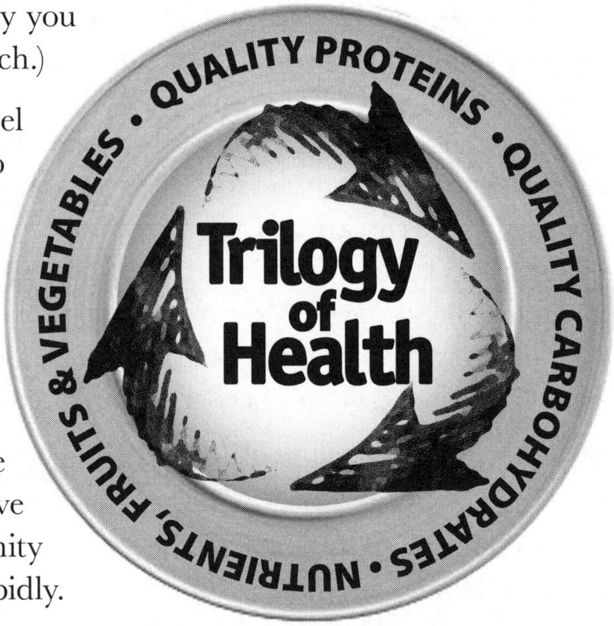

DESSERTS

You must give up desserts forver! Haaahaaaha! Cries the evil laugh!

Ah, desserts. Everyone's favorite topic. If you listen to the evil laugh, how much fun would life be? You can have desserts. In fact, you should if you are so inclined, but in moderation. However, desserts can be the bane of your fat-loss efforts if you choose the wrong kinds or opt for double-sized portions. Overindulging in desserts will oversize your waistline.

Some desserts contain as much as 80 grams of fat and over 1,000 calories in a single serving. That is more than a day's worth of fat and about half the caloric intake you need in a day. It is easy to see how overindulging, or making wrong choices, can pack on the pounds! Where does this leave you? You need to be selective about when and what you have for dessert.

To be successful in your goals you must

- choose appropriately.
- limit frequency.
- limit quantity.

You say that you want dessert more often than a few times a year; I do, too. On a more regular basis, but still being selective, you can have desserts that do not contain a gazillion calories and grams of fat. For example,

DESSERT EXAMPLES

	Calories	Grams of Fat
Fruit	35 - 105	0
Sherbet	140	1
Ice cream (no fat)	120	0
Ice cream (4oz)	200 - 350	10-25
Chocolate wall	1883	71

an angel food cake cup with fresh fruit contains only 150 calories and no fat; it also provides a fruit serving for the day. You can also have a fruit dish with a small scoop of sorbet or low-fat ice cream. Try soy ice cream; it's better for you and just as tasty. Okay, so you want that double-chocolate, decadent mousse cake. Go ahead, but ask for a half slice or share a piece with a friend or two. Just think of how great you will feel at the end of the day knowing that you have followed your plan, exercised, eaten healthful foods, and shared a delectable dessert with someone special. The only thing that you will miss is the guilt. The *BetterBody BetterLife* philosophy is to eat in a healthful manner, not to make life boring or restrictive.

Desserts can be a part of your life when chosen with awareness.

- Moderation is good. Excess is bad!
- Moderation, balance, and variety.

THE EDUCATED CONSUMER

Although you needn't count calories per se, you need to understand calories and how they vary by food and product. Your knowledge will help you make educated decisions and choices. When you are at a restaurant deciding which meal to order or in a market shopping for food, you need to know which foods are the healthy choices. Even the same products from different companies can be dramatically different in total fat and calories.

Nearly every food product has a nutrition label on it somewhere. What do the words and numbers on that label mean? Which ones are important? They are all important, but some are key. You do not need a Ph.D. to understand a nutrition label. You simply need to know how to decipher which food products to pass by and which to take home with you.

The United States Food and Drug Administration (FDA) requires that most processed food products bear a nutrition label. Among other things, the label information shows how the product measures up against the government's Dietary Reference Intakes (DRIs) of nutrients and some vitamins and minerals. The DRI is the amount of protein, carbohydrate, dietary fat, or other nutrients generally considered appropriate for people of different ages, sexes, and activity levels. The amounts of nutrients on nutritional labels are expressed as a percentage of the DRI provided in one serving, based on an adult diet of 2,000 calories per day. Nutritional labels are a great reference tool to use when shopping and preparing meals, but 2,000 calories a day won't promote body-fat loss in most people. Also, note that the DRI for total fat in a 2,000-calorie diet is 65 grams. That amount is high for those in a body-fat reduction program.

Learn to read labels and understand the nutritional value of food. Doing so will make you keenly aware of the benefits of your choices. Read labels not to learn to count calories, but to become aware of the benefit of one choice over another. Savvy shoppers make wise decisions about nutritional choices while minimizing sacrifices.

INGREDIENTS

Ingredients are listed on the nutrition label. You may not count calories, but you need to be smart about the ingredients in the food you eat. Ingredients are listed in order of quantity from most to least. The first few ingredients listed should be natural foods such as wheat, tomatoes, or water. The first ingredients should not be high fructose corn syrup, corn syrup, hydrogenated, bleached, sugar, or salt. If possible avoid these ingredients altogether, but if they are in your food, make sure such

ON THE LABEL

LOOK:
- Is it the same size as what you need?
- How many servings are in the package?
- Note the number of calories.

AFTER PREPARATION:
- Is it higher in fat or calories?
- Choose products low in total fat, especially those low in saturated fat.

LIMIT
- Cholesterol, sodium, total fat, and saturated fat as much as possible.

ingredients are the last on the list. There is always a healthy alternative to any food. Learning what is the best option will be a learning curve. It is up to you to determine the best foods to buy and eat. Nobody else will do it for you. Even foods advertised as healthy choices are often not very healthy. It is your responsibility to read the labels and ingredients and determine if a food is a good choice. If you are unsure if an ingredient is a good or bad food, Google the ingredient. An educated consumer is only a click away.

VITAMINS, MINERALS, AND SUPPLEMENTS

Those who eat a complete and balanced diet do not need to add supplements to their diets. A complete, balanced, and varied diet — such as that recommended in the *BetterBody BetterLife* plan — provides sufficient amounts of vitamins, minerals, and nutrients from natural foods. Those eating in a healthful manner can easily obtain the nutrients they need daily. In levels below that, however, a person can become nutrient deficient. At the other extreme, excessive levels are toxic. Large doses of supplements can cause short-term, long-term, and even permanent damage to the body's organs and structure.

Therefore, when choosing a vitamin supplement, be very cautious. More is not necessarily better. The average, healthy, fit, active person who eats a well-balanced diet does not need extra supplements. Those who have extraordinary needs should consult a physician, or nutritionist, for specific advice. Those with medical issues, pregnant women, or nursing women may also have special needs. If you chose to take a supplement, do not take one that offers much more than 100 percent of the average daily value (for an adult), unless directed to do so by a health professional. Don't fall prey to the promotions that claim you need megadoses of anything.

FAT-FREE FOODS

Although many products tout "fat-free" on the label, you can't eat all you want of them. You may or may not be making a better choice when you eat a fat-free brownie instead of a traditional one. The fat-free brownie still has calories from carbohydrates (sugar). Often, it has even more calories than the traditional food because extra sugars are added for flavor. So pay attention to labels and nutritional content and make the most appropriate choices for your goals. The choice may not be which brownie to eat, but whether you should eat one at all.

As you can see, this program is about moderation and making healthful choices most often. It is not difficult, and you can still enjoy many of the comforting and pleasurable foods that you currently enjoy. The difference lies in moderation, portion size, and food choices. To manage your health, be conscious of the foods you choose. Otherwise, your life will be a never-ending battle of yo-yo dieting.

"Behave so the aroma of your actions may enhance the general sweetness of the atmosphere."

HENRY DAVID THOREAU

Chapter Twenty-Two

THE NUTRITION PLAN

Would you like a plan that is easy to follow for body-fat loss? It is time to put your knowledge to use and construct that plan. By now, you should have a good grasp of the fundamentals of nutrition. The plan you construct will form the foundation you need to become healthy so you can achieve physical freedom and a healthful future.

As you construct your plan, always remember our key phrases:

Moderation is good. Excess is bad.
Moderation, balance, and variety

BODY-FAT LOSS

To lose body fat and reduce your weight, you must consume fewer calories than you expend through metabolic, muscular, and digestive activities. You put on body fat slowly over a long period of time; it needs to come off the same way. One pound of fat equals 3,500 calories; therefore, to lose 1 pound of body fat, you need to burn and reduce calories to achieve a 3,500-calorie deficit. If you divide 3,500 by 7 (days), the deficit equals 500 calories per day. If your goal for weight loss is to lose 2 pounds of body fat per week, on average, then you need to reduce your calorie intake by 500 daily and increase your metabolism through fitness conditioning to burn an additional 500 calories a day. Those measures result in a total calorie deficit of 1,000 calories a day, or 7,000 calories a week. A 7,000-calorie deficit equals 2 pounds of body fat lost each week. It's a numbers thing!

You will notice at times that you are losing more than 2 pounds a week. This is especially true when you first start a fitness plan. When you fill your body with healthy, nourishing food and water, an early, dramatic weight loss is likely. It's mostly water. If you usually eat a lot of processed foods and then you switch to natural foods, your physiology changes from the dramatic reduction in your intake of sodium, sugars, chemicals, and fat. Processed foods are generally loaded with sodium (salt) and chemical additives with unpronounceable names. Salt and additives cause your body to retain water. Early in a program, your body loses that water. This is another reason why you need four bottles of water a day. After your body adjusts to the changes and levels out, long-term success depends on a net reduction in calories from nutrition and exercise.

Note: If your calorie requirements equal 2,500 calories per day, but you are consuming 4,000 calories a day, then reducing your intake by 1,000 calories will only slow the rate of body-fat gain. You will still be consuming 3,000 calories, or 500 calories more than your body needs per day. If you are consuming an excessive number of calories, reduce your calorie consumption to 500 calories less than your body needs and increase your activity by an equal amount. In this example, limit calories to 2,000 a day; then increase your metabolism by 500 calories a day with an active lifestyle and exercise conditioning. This will net a deficit of 1,000 calories and produce a 2-pound-a-week body-fat loss.

A female with an average frame at a healthy weight (5'4" and 125 pounds) utilizes approximately 2,300 calories a day. An average male (5'8" and 170 pounds) utilizes about 2,600 calories a day. As a result, an average female who needs to lose body fat will limit calorie consumption to 1,800 per day; an average male, to 2,100. Since we are not counting calories, this exercise merely gives you an idea about how your body works. You may need to eat more or less, depending on your body type. Learn your body's signals. It will tell you when you need to make adjustments. At no time should you consume fewer than 1,500 calories a day. Less is dangerous because you cannot get the proper nutrients.

If you want to count calories, by all means do so. I encourage you to be a calorie- and fat-gram counter. You will better understand your eating strengths and weaknesses, but counting is not required for success. When choosing foods, read labels and consider how food choices affect your plan. Eat sensibly! If the average woman consumes 1,200 calories in a single meal, then she has only 600 calories left for the rest of the day. That does not give her much chance for success. A large bag of potato chips or a dessert containing 600 or 700 calories can put you over your calorie-maximum for the day.

Note: I wish that I could tell you exactly how many calories to eat. Since I don't know your frame, age, weight, body-fat percentage, usual diet, lifestyle, exercise regimen, or medical history, I can't give you an exact number. The estimates of 1,800 to 2,100 calories a day are simply an average range. You must determine where in that range you should be. The best way is to listen to your body and let the results of your efforts tell you how you are doing. Make honest assessments of your results, body type, and lifestyle; then adjust your plan accordingly.

GRAMS OF FAT

Unsaturated fat is good for you in small amounts, and saturated fat is not. Therefore, the fat that you consume should be mostly unsaturated. Women should limit dietary fat consumption to 40 grams per day. That equates to about 20 percent of the calories in a woman's weight-loss diet of 1,800 calories daily. An average man should limit fat to 46 grams per day.

WHAT TO EAT EVERY DAY

- Vegetables
  5 or more servings a day
- Fruit
  4 or more servings a day
- Quality carbohydrates - Whole-grain
  3 servings a day
- Milk and dairy
  Limit to 2 servings a day
- Protein - Lean and clean
  Beans, nuts, seeds, soy, or complementary vegetables
  Limit meat to 1 serving a day
- Sweets and fats
  Avoid or limit as much as possible
  Choose unsaturated fats most often.

Some will argue that 20 percent of caloric intake a day from fat is low; after all, the U.S. government allows almost 30 percent, or up to 65 grams for a 2,000-calorie diet. However, when body-fat reduction is the goal, calories and fat must be limited. The government's suggestion is generous even for a weight-maintenance program; that much fat certainly will not cause body-fat loss in most people. Is 40 grams of fat a day a strict rule? No. It is a guideline. Remember, body management is an average of all of your efforts. Some days you will consume more, and some, less. Strive for progress, not perfection. When you have reached your body-fat goal, you can then adjust to a maintenance plan.

Change your thoughts and you change your world.

NORMAN VINCENT PEALE

MEN

- Limit calories from 1,800 to 2,400 per day.
- Limit fat to 46 grams per day.
- Limit saturated (bad) fat to 12 grams (part of total fat) per day.
- Eat a well-balanced diet from all of the food categories.
- Choose low-fat, low-calorie options when possible.

WOMEN

- Limit calories from 1,800 to 2,100 per day.
- Limit fat to 40 grams per day.
- Limit saturated (bad) fat to 11 grams (part of total fat) per day.
- Eat a well-balanced diet from all of the food categories.
- Choose low-fat, low-calorie options when possible.

Chapter Twenty-Three

THE NEXT STEP

We are almost there. I know I've included a lot of information here. You may need some time to learn all the details. I promise, in time healthy eating will become second nature. Change your habits and change your life, but life changes don't happen overnight. In this plan and in life, your success is about progress, not perfection. Nobody is perfect, so expecting perfection is unreasonable. When you fail — and you will at times — learn from your failures. When you succeed — and you will — repeat your successes and feel brilliant about them. Be grateful for failure and success because both are part of success. Olympic athletes repeatedly fail as they master their sports; actors and models go to countless auditions before they land a job; and toddlers stumble and bump for months until they learn to walk.

How many times would you let your child fall before saying, "That's enough, pumpkin. You don't need to walk." It wouldn't happen. Children try and try until they get it right. Parents offer repeated help and encouragement until their children learn to walk on their own. As adults we are less patient. We often stop after a couple of tries of something new, thinking the payoff may not be worth the effort. Your health is worth some effort! Health, fitness, and weight loss are musts!

Those who are most successful constantly evaluate their efforts, failures, and successes. Life and learning are a process, and part of that process is finding your weaknesses and strengths. One of the best ways to find your ups and downs is to record and review what you do. You may have been keeping a journal for a while; if not, now is the time to begin. Skip this step ONLY if you plan to fail. Your journal is your map, your record, and your best tool. In your journal, you will plan, record, and evaluate your day. Remember how you felt when you looked at the photos you took of yourself in a bathing suit? The experience was enlightening and revealing, wasn't it? Your journal will give you that kind of insight. It will give you a snapshot of your day. You will see at a glance if your eating habits are impressive or in need of intervention. You will quickly find the good and bad patterns in your fitness routines, or lack thereof. And if you look carefully, you will find excuses that need to be eliminated and patterns that need to be improved.

Grab your *BetterBody BetterLife* Journal and record your new knowledge and information. Go to the *Dreams to Goals* ***worksheet*** on page 53 and write the nutritional criteria that you will use.

For example:
I will limit fat to 40 grams per day and calories to 1,800 per day.
I will plan each meal so that it's balanced with green nutrients, protein, and quality carbohydrates.
I will eat 3 balanced meals and 2 midmeals each day.
I will drink 4 bottles of water each day.

PLANNING YOUR DAY

About 70 percent of Americans do not plan dinner until after 4 P.M. The result is often not a quality meal but supersized fast foods, pizza; or frozen dinners. With habits like those of the masses, you will be like the masses.

Open to the first day in your journal. Review the format and start filling out the basic information. Next, plan your meals for the day. Fill in the types of food you plan to have for breakfast, midmeals, lunch, and dinner. This plan will take the guesswork out of your day. The *BetterBody BetterLife Journal* is small and portable so you can keep it with you. Fill in the required information and make notes throughout the day. If you rely on your memory and try to fill in your journal at the end of the day, you will paint a rosier picture. You will forget foods you ate and overestimate the time you exercised.

Make a realistic plan for each day and then follow the plan. Life will get in the way from time to time, but interruptions shouldn't occur too often. If you find that you are not making or following your plan, then evaluate the reasons and change your patterns. If your first change doesn't work, change your patterns again. If your second change doesn't work, change them again. How many times will you change your patterns and try something new? Until you find the pattern that works for you! At the end of the day, review your efforts and plan the next day, learning from your accomplishments and failures.

Plan
- when you will eat
- what you will eat
- where you will eat
- how you will get your meals
- why you will eat

Don't leave anything to chance.
Plan it and make it happen!

RECORD IT

Every time you put something into your mouth, record what you ate or drank in your journal. Record coffee, crackers, candy, lunch, dinner, water, and anything else you consume, whether it was planned or not. Most people consume much more food than they remember or realize – sometimes out of habit, sometimes out boredom, sometimes out of emotional need. If you wish, you can calculate the number of fat grams and calories you consumed for the day, but you don't have to if you are eating quality, natural foods in moderate portions.

REVIEW THE DAY

At the end of the day, after you have recorded everything that you consumed throughout the day, you can assess how you did and decide what you can do the next day to improve. Did you eat the meals that you planned? Did you go to the candy machine…often? Did you exercise? Did you keep your general activity level up? Did you drink four bottles of water?

From reviewing your journal, you can learn to avoid situations that promote snacking and cheating. For example, if cookies and pastries are always available during your coffee break at the office, you can make a conscious choice. Either you can stay away ("out of sight, out of mind") or you can take a good snack with you from home to eat at that time. The easiest way to stay on course is to avoid situations that can lead you astray. A salesperson would not leave a cash register drawer open to tempt a passerby; why should you keep processed junk food close by? You can be proactive and request that healthful foods be available at conferences or in the break room. I bet that others who work with you will appreciate better choices, too.

After you have reviewed your day, jot some notes about how you feel you did and how you might improve. Write a short summary of your day. Was it a great day? Or a day when you could have done better? Record what prevented you from sticking to your plan and record what helped you. Then plan the next day.

As with any learning experience, keeping your journal may seem cumbersome at first, but in a short time, the record keeping becomes natural and easy. When trying diet after diet plan, have you ever kept a journal? Probably not, or maybe you stopped for some reason. Change your pattern and change your life. If you create healthy habits and a healthy lifestyle, then you can be successful for life. Then the opposite happens; once you develop healthy living habits, your body will instinctively tell you to stop eating garbage if you deviate from the plan.

"You may never know what results come of your action, but if you do nothing there will be no result."

MAHATMA GANDHI

Chapter Twenty-Four

NUTRITION PLAN EXAMPLES

On the following pages, you will find five daily menu plans with examples of healthful meals and midmeals. Use these to plan and to create your own daily menu. Remember to read the labels of the food products you purchase and the premade meals you eat. Healthy nutrition is easy, once you know the fundamentals.

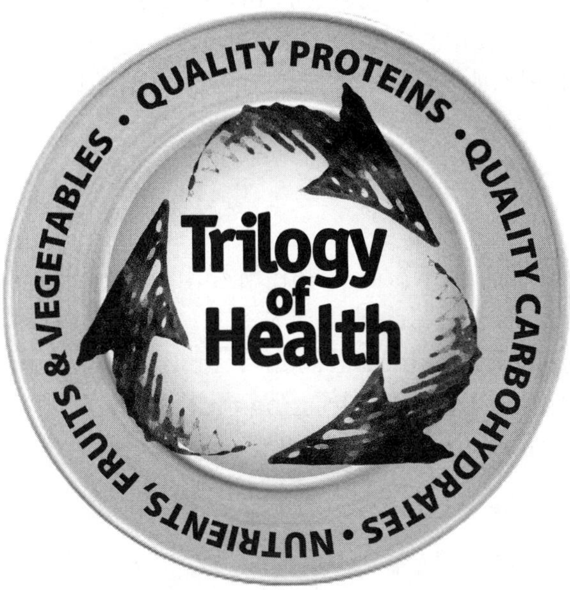

BALANCE YOUR PLATE WITH A WIDE VARIETY OF HEALTHY UNPROCESSED FOOD.

Use the following menu examples as a guide and choose foods that you like.

MENU EXAMPLE 1

Powerfest	Hot or cold cereal with a fruit cup
Midmeal snack	Cottage cheese with fruit
Lunch	Roasted veggie wrap and side garden salad
Midmeal snack	Pretzels and almonds (1/2 cup)
Dinner	Vegetable stir-fry with tofu, chicken, or fish

MENU EXAMPLE 2

Powerfest	Fruit smoothie with soy milk
Midmeal snack	Whole-grain toast (1 slice) with peanut butter and fruit spread
Lunch	Turkey with lettuce, tomato, and cheese pita or sandwich with baked chips
Midmeal snack	Carrots and celery sticks
Dinner	Grilled fish, bruschetta, and sautéed spinach

MENU EXAMPLE 3

Powerfest	Breakfast burrito (1 egg, vegetables and cheese), and orange juice
Midmeal snack	Fruit cup
Lunch	Pasta salad with veggies and fruit
Midmeal snack	Unsalted blue corn tortilla chips and salsa
Dinner	Grilled sirloin, sweet potato, and grilled asparagus

MENU EXAMPLE 4

Powerfest	French toast (whole-grain bread) with berries
Midmeal snack	Almonds and dried fruit
Lunch	Broth soup, half sandwich, and mixed green side salad with the dressing on the side
Midmeal snack	Popcorn (salt-free and butter-free)
Dinner	Southwest beans and rice with grilled peppers

MENU EXAMPLE 5

Powerfest	Wheat pancakes and bananas
Midmeal snack	Fat-free yogurt with fresh fruit
Lunch	Vegetables with rice in curry sauce
Midmeal snack	Trail mix (1/4 cup)
Dinner	Stuffed green bell pepper, spinach salad, and corn on the cob

WITH ALL MEALS

- Drink a glass of water with all meals (8 cups a day or 4 water bottles).
- Meals can include tea or coffee, but go very easy on the sugar and milk.
- Soda and alcoholic drinks are calorie dense and should be avoided or limited.

DESSERT IDEAS

- Angel food cup with fruit
- Fruit and sorbet
- Dairy-free ice cream (soy frozen dessert)
- Fruit smoothie made with soy milk
- Banana split with dairy-free ice cream and nuts
- Or make any dessert with a lower-calorie recipe or share a dessert with someone special.

Knowing is not enough, we must apply.
Willing is not enough, we must do.

JOHANN VON GOETHE

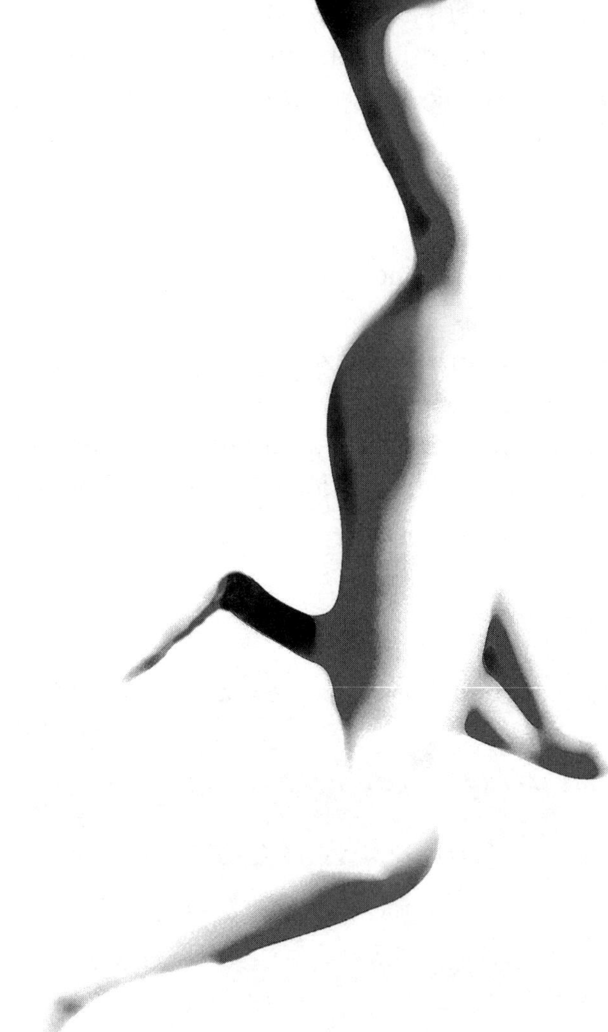

Section Three

Fitness for a Fabulous Body

Chapter Twenty-Five

FIT FEELS GOOD

Would you like to feel extraordinary every day?
Would you like to have a ton of energy all day long?
Do you want to look fabulous at the beach?

You can have it all and it's easy! You understand the importance of healthy nutrition and how good food choices create the foundation of your life. Now you will learn to build a temple on that foundation. What? You don't think of your body as a temple? It is. Your body is the most beautiful sculpture in the world. The greatest part: you can continue to sculpt your body until you get the masterpiece of your dreams. You are beautiful and you are amazing! Think of yourself as a mythological goddess or god in the making.

You can create a breathtaking physique. It's totally within your reach and control. Fitness conditioning, a.k.a. exercise, will turn your body into a fat-burning machine. The conversion happens when you replace body fat with toned muscle. Cardiovascular conditioning and muscle toning are essential for a full and healthy life. They have numerous benefits. They help you feel, think, look, and live better. The benefits are internal as well as external. Stronger muscles, a leaner physique, better heart and lung function, lower cholesterol, lower weight, and less body fat are just a few.

DO YOU DREAD EXERCISE?

For many, taking time out of a busy day to exercise is not an appealing idea. Many people are not motivated to exercise, so they easily brush it aside. Like many people, some days I need to create motivation or coerce myself into exercise. But every time I finish, I'm so glad I exercised. The days when I want to work out the least are the days I usually feel the best when I'm done. For the rest of the day after your workout, you will feel great. You will know that you are moving toward a healthier and happier you.

Do you agree that every day you wake up and look down at the ground is a great day? If you don't think so, try missing just one of them. Every day starts the same way for me. I sit down with a glass of fresh orange juice and read for a few minutes while my body transitions from sleep to conscious functioning. Then I work out. When I exercise, I celebrate another day of living. I take care of my body because I value having one more day to look into the eyes of my beautiful wife and to see my daughter's captivating smile. Most days I look forward to fitness conditioning because having the ability to exercise is a gift. I meet many people who do not have the gift of health, and most of them wish they had their health again. If you do not think exercise is a gift, go to YouTube.com and search for "Team Hoyt." Watch a video of this amazing father and son. You will cry and you will be thankful for everything in your life.

YOUR BEST ALLY

The *Trilogy of Health* philosophy of proper nutrition, cardiovascular conditioning, and muscle toning becomes more and more important with age; improving your physical condition at every age is vital to an active and vibrant life. If you neglect your home for long, it will become dilapidated and require difficult repairs. If the human body is neglected for long, it becomes weak, frail, and sick. It falls into ruins and collapses. Like a neglected building, it becomes a shell of its prior self, and it fails much sooner than it should. Regular health maintenance staves off a failing and weak body. To keep your body strong and resistant to the effects of age, gravity, and illness, make the *Trilogy of Health* a daily ritual. A strong, healthy body throughout life will be your best ally.

The first component, proper nutrition, gives your body the fuel it needs to orchestrate the other two components, cardiovascular conditioning and muscle toning. Achieving the body you dream of is as straightforward as attending to all three components. Although the three components are distinct, cardiovascular conditioning and muscle toning complement each other closely, and they depend on proper nutrition for success.

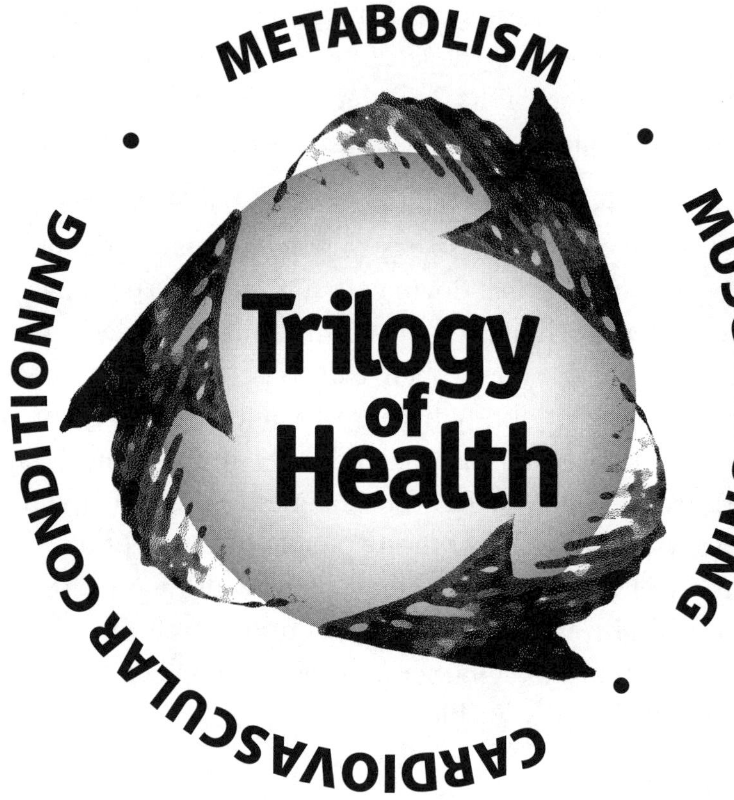

Let me describe the ultimate physique:

A body with a healthy body-fat percentage.
A look that states, "I'm fit. I love life and who I am."
A body that feels great with energy and balance.

You do not have to look like a fitness model to be healthy. An active person who exercises, eats properly, and maintains a physique that is neither too thin nor too fat is an icon of health, even without the six-pack abs. Of course, if you desire a muscular six pack, that goal is within your reach with this program.

When you implement the *Trilogy of Health*, a synergistic effect takes place. Synergy is when the sum of the parts equals more than the whole. For example, 2+2 = 7. When the components of the *Trilogy of Health* are synchronized, the three components complement and compound one another's effects, causing a greater result. Synergy is the key to liberation from dieting. The *Trilogy of Health* explains how our bodies are designed, and it defines the only proven way to maintain a healthy physique for the duration of your life.

WHAT TO EXPECT

In this section, we will discuss why it's important to improve your cardiovascular ability and to tone your muscle structure. You will also learn how to achieve great results in the most efficient way possible.

A complete fitness routine will

- reduce fatigue
- reduce stress, anxiety, and depression
- reduce body fat
- increase mobility
- increase strength
- increase flexibility
- increase energy
- increase endurance
- increase brain cells
- increase muscle tone and definition
- improve sex
- promote healthy bones
- manage weight naturally
- lower risk factors for disease
- promote the health of the heart and arteries

Imagine what you can do with more energy, mobility, and strength. How will you feel when you look in the mirror and see a fit, toned, and tight body? If you don't work at becoming strong and healthy, your body will literally waste away. Just look at all the elderly people who are withered shells of what they once were. Age doesn't have to be that way.

In recent studies, scientists have learned that there is a correlation between exercising and brain-cell production. Remember all the brains cells you destroyed in your wilder days? Those that are lost are long gone, but you can replace them with new ones. Not only will you get in better physical shape, but you will get smarter as well.

WHAT IS FITNESS CONDITIONING?

Cardiovascular conditioning is the process of performing any endurance activity (e.g. walking, jogging, or aerobics) that will raise your heart rate, increase your breathing rate and metabolism, and burn additional calories.

Muscle toning is the process of performing any activity that increases muscular strength with resistance training. Muscle toning enhances one's ability to perform general or specific activities, increases the body's metabolic rate, and reduces body fat.

Get maximum results while minimizing the effort. Don't confuse getting maximal results while minimizing effort with a "no-effort" plan. This is not a "quick fix" plan, and effort does equal results. What you put in, you get out. This is a "permanent fix" plan and a lifestyle plan. The results depend on your goals and your resolve to achieve those goals. Your success will be a direct result of how disciplined you are in carrying out the daily steps of a healthy lifestyle. The beautiful part of this plan is that it helps you work smarter, not harder. Getting maximal results while minimizing effort means getting the most out of what you do and performing the task using the most efficient method.

Imagine this: You're standing in front of a fence and you need to get to the other side. What will you do?

Would you ...climb over the fence?
...run through the fence?
...walk to the gate just a few steps to the side?

Most people would choose to walk to the gate. That approach is the most efficient way to accomplish the task. You assess the obstacle, the fence, and then decide to walk to the gate and go through. That strategy gets you to your destination with the least amount of effort, and it achieves your goal of getting to the other side.

BECOME ACTIVE

In this era of remote controls and automatic everything, many conveniences make life easier. The more your life is automated, the fewer chances you have to burn calories. The first step toward a healthy and fit body is to find plenty of ways to burn calories. The idea is to assist your body in staying fit naturally through everyday occurrences. Anything you do that requires physical effort burns additional calories and raises your metabolism.

I frequently see people doing anything, and everything, to avoid something that requires the smallest amount of energy. Sometimes people go to great lengths just to avoid walking a few extra yards or getting out of a car. How many times have you seen someone driving around the mall parking lot, circling the lanes four or five times to find a closer parking spot? Or have you seen a driver moving a car forward and backward to get closer to a mailbox to avoid getting out of the car and walking a couple of feet?

HOW PHYSICALLY ACTIVE IS THE U.S. POPULATION?

A recent study showed that only 22 percent of adults get the recommended regular physical activity (5 times a week for at least 30 minutes) of any intensity during leisure time. About 15 percent get the recommended amount of vigorous activity (3 times a week for at least 20 minutes). About 25 percent of adults claim they do no physical activity at all in their leisure time.

What will happen if you become a little more active?

You will burn a few more calories.

What will happen if you become a lot more active?

You will burn a lot more calories.

Losing body fat depends on consistently raising your metabolism and burning more calories than you need. It's simple mathematics. Being a couch potato only makes you look like a potato. Where do you think that phrase came from?

To lose body fat, you must first raise your metabolism throughout the day. Incorporating small, even seemingly inconsequential activities into your day can result in an overall increase in metabolism. You may burn only a few extra calories at a time, but when added together, the increase is significant. An additional 10 calories here and 20 calories there can add up to several hundred a day, or more. Add to your day as many activities in the next list as you can. Then see how many additional calories you burn even before you exercise.

Calorie-Burning Activities

Activity	Calories Used*
Use the stairs (per story)	25
Walk to the mailbox	20
Park in the far lot and walk	30
A 10-minute walk (brisk)	75
Washing your car	150
Playing with children (30 minutes)	200
Raking (30 minutes)	190
Gardening/yard work (30 minutes)	170
Dancing (30 minutes)	180
Playing volleyball or badminton (30 minutes)	300
Yoga (30 minutes)	150

Compare to

Sleeping (30 minutes)	32
Watching TV (30 minutes)	35

* These figures are averages. The actual number of calories burned depends on your weight, your fitness, and the effort you expend. Results will vary.

Remember, every deficit of 3,500 calories will result in 1 pound of lost body fat. The little activities that make you less idle will burn more calories, so you can lose body fat more easily and more quickly. Walk instead of drive any time you can. Get out of your car and walk into a building instead of using the drive-through. Take the stairs instead of the elevator. Walk or jog with your dog; your dog will love you for it. Walk other people's dogs and get paid for it. Why not save money losing weight? Do your own yard work. The lawn and your body will look great. (Sitting on a riding lawn mower doesn't count.) I have a friend who is past age 70; he still pushes his little mower as if mowing were an Olympic sport. Do some housecleaning with extra vigor. Turn on your stereo and clean with zest; you have to do the chores anyway. Play with your children: play ball, tag, or hide-and-seek. Catch lightning bugs (but be sure to let them go). Build better relationships and a better body. All of these measures will help your body become better at burning calories. Do you get the idea? Get off the couch and do something — anything. The couch is the malediction of a fit body. The "body fat-devil" is your couch; it will keep you in his clutches like an 800-pound gorilla. Become more active overall, and your body will become and stay lean.

Becoming more active increases your endurance. An active body develops a higher resting metabolism and burns additional calories, which helps you become and stay naturally lean.

"We are all faced with a series of great opportunities brilliantly disguised as impossible situations."

CHARLES R. SWINDOLL

Chapter Twenty-Six

CARDIOVASCULAR CONDITIONING

In addition to becoming more active throughout the day, we also need to condition the body. Cardiovascular conditioning is any endurance activity that increases breathing rate, heart rate, and metabolism, thereby burning additional calories. Such increases are achieved best through specific and dynamic "cardiovascular conditioning workouts," also known as "cardio workouts." Workouts require exercising at specific levels for minimum amounts of time. This isn't as technical as it sounds. Simply stated, it's a minimum of 20 minutes of cardiovascular conditioning performed three times a week.

In those 20 minutes, you will train and condition your body to perform at a higher than normal — or dynamic — level. All of the body's systems — cardiovascular, musculoskeletal, respiratory, nervous, and endocrine — will benefit from this conditioning. When you exercise at a higher than normal level, the body produces many chemicals, and many chemical reactions take place. You may feel some of those chemical changes as a "cardio high." Cardiovascular conditioning sessions benefit the body by developing a higher endurance level and by making the whole body fit, including organs. Cardiovascular conditioning gives your body some physical strength but more important, it gives you higher levels of energy and endurance to complete everyday tasks more easily. That improves your ability to climb stairs, carry groceries, play with children, and deal with the occasional emergency. A fit and healthy body has a lower resting heart rate. That means that the heart works less to produce the same results. Think of it as a low-mileage heart. But wait! There's more! Cardiovascular conditioning promotes a higher resting metabolism so that your body burns more calories, even when at rest.

Perform your cardio workout three times a week. A multitude of activities qualify as cardio workouts. Pick something that you enjoy and you will be more likely to stick with your cardio exercise program. If you change your cardio workout frequently, you will never be bored and you will get better results.

SOME CARDIO ACTIVITIES TO CONSIDER		
Aerobics classes	Jogging	Rollerblading
Badminton	Jumping jacks	Skiing
Basketball	Jumping rope	Spinning
Bicycling	Kayaking	Squash
Brisk walking	Kickboxing	Swimming
Dancing	Power yoga	Tennis
Hiking	Racquetball	Volleyball

THE CARDIO PLAN

This is a simple cardio plan with only 20 minutes of dynamic exercise. The total time is only 30 minutes when you include warmup, cool down, and stretching.

Start:

3-minute warmup

Then:

20 minutes of dynamic cardiovascular conditioning

End:

2 minutes of cool down

5 minutes of stretching

That's it! That doesn't sound hard, does it?

WARMUP

The 3-minute warmup notifies your body that you are about to start exercising. Think of it as a big, red flag. It signals your body to begin its chemical changes, and it reduces your chances for injury.

WARMUP AT A LEVEL-5

On a scale of 1 to 10 (where 1 is loafing around and 10 is an all-out effort), your 3-minute warmup should achieve a level-5. For example, this may be at the cardio level of a brisk walk or an easy jog. This depends on your physical condition and should be at your level-5 for 3 minutes.

20-MINUTE CARDIOVASCULAR CONDITIONING SESSION

During the 20-minute session, you should exercise in 4-minute cycles. In each cycle, increase the pace in each of the first 3 minutes. During the fourth minute of the cycle, slow to a level-5 intensity. (See chart on next page)

COOL DOWN AND STRETCHING

After you have completed your 20 minutes of dynamic cardiovascular conditioning, you must cool down properly. Slowly bring your body back down to an exertion level-4 and continue at this pace for 2 minutes. The cool down allows your body to recognize that the work is over.

After your workout, stretch the muscles you exercised. Never bounce while stretching. Ask a personal trainer or professional to teach you how to stretch properly.

To Illustrate: Warmup at level-5 for 3 minutes. Then, start your dynamic cardio session. In the first minute of your dynamic cardio session, increase to a level-6. Then, increase your output by 1 level for each minute. At the fourth minute, reduce your intensity back to level-5. At the fifth minute, increase your output for each of the next 3 minutes by one level. Then, slow back to a level-5.

At the sixteenth minute, reduce to your level-6 instead of a level-5. In each of the next minutes, increase the intensity by one level. The seventeenth minute should be your level-7, and the eighteenth minute will be your level-8. For the last 2 minutes, go for an all-out effort. At the nineteenth minute, increase your energy output to a level-9, and for the twentieth minute (the last minute), take your effort to its maximum, a level-10. (See maximum heart rate on page 217.)

INTERVAL TRAINING CHART

Stepping up your exertion level and then slowing down is called interval training. If at some point you feel that you are overdoing it, back off the pace a little and then increase the pace again after a minute or two. It is far better to slow down than to injure yourself. A pulled muscle can keep you out of commission for several weeks. Then how much exercising will you be doing? Forget the "no pain, no gain" mantra. However, you should be pushing yourself to a level that is challenging and difficult; otherwise the benefits will be nil. You should keep your conditioning sessions to a level that is safe for you. You are not a professional athlete; don't think that you have to train like one.

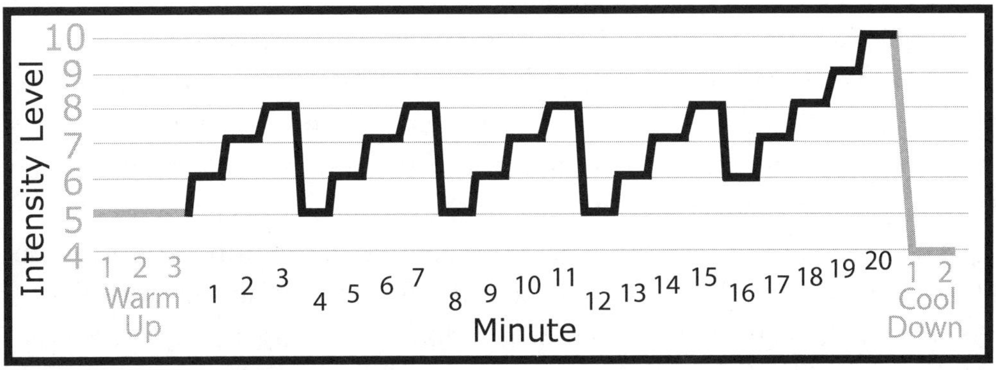

COOL DOWN

Now slow down gradually from level-10 to a cool down pace of level-4. DO NOT skip the cool down at the end. Your body needs to know that you are finished. This period allows the body to gradually slow down, permitting your muscles, circulatory system, and respiratory system time to cycle down and allowing chemical fluctuations to begin to stabilize. Skipping the cool down is like racing a car at breakneck speed and then slamming on the brakes. It creates unwarranted stress and damage to systems.

At the end of your 20-minute conditioning session (you don't need to stop at 20 minutes), slow down to a cooling pace and continue at this reduced pace for 2 more minutes. Continue at a cool-down pace for several additional minutes or longer until your body cycles down completely. The cooling pace should be 50 percent (level-4) of the highest normal interval pace (level-8) during your training. It's important to keep moving, but at a reduced pace, to give your muscles time to cool down and to signal your muscles that the high demands are completed.

It is also very important to stretch all the muscles that you have just conditioned. For the next 5 minutes, you will need to loosen your muscles with stretching. When you exercise, lactic acid builds up in the exercised and stressed muscles; it can lead to excess muscle soreness if you do not stretch. You should stretch all of your muscles, especially your hamstrings (back of the thighs), back, and shoulders.

I prefer and recommend cardiovascular equipment that trains the upper and lower body, such as elliptical machines with arm row or rowing machines. These types of machines offer a better workout at lower speeds and help to tone the whole body. You need not, however, work on a machine. Choose any exercise that you enjoy. Swimming is the best cardio workout you can get. You can get dynamic cardiovascular conditioning with sports, such as volleyball, racquetball, or tennis. You may need more time to get the same result because of the lower and intermittent energy expenditure. I participate in different sports in adult leagues and community programs to get some of my cardiovascular conditioning. I look forward to playing Tuesday night volleyball at the local school (noncompetition fun league), playing softball in the summer, and swimming and playing racquetball throughout the winter. These activities help to make staying healthy fun, and they allow me to get together with friends. Cardiovascular conditioning

Note: If you're starting for the first time or starting again after a long period of not exercising, start off slowly. If you stress your body too quickly, your body will retaliate with slow progress, excessive soreness, and perhaps even an injury. Even if you have exercised regularly in the past, do not expect to pick up where you left off last. If you do, you'll regret your decision for several days. Start with 2 weeks of low to moderate training. If you are currently sedentary and have little exercise experience, then I recommend that you simply walk 3 times a week for 30 minutes at a level-5 or level-6. If you cannot walk for 30 minutes, start off with fewer minutes, gradually increasing the duration to 30 minutes; then move on with the rest of the plan. You need to make your body aware of your new exercise program; if you don't, you will greatly increase your risk of injury.

can also be accomplished with Sunday afternoon activities that include your spouse, children, and pets. Take the family hiking, biking, or swimming.

LIFE GETS EASIER

In only 30 minutes per day, you will burn 100 to 500 calories, depending on your activity intensity, your weight, your age, and your fitness level. Your metabolism will remain elevated, and you will burn additional calories for the next few hours.

Cardio offers benefits in addition to the health of your organs, muscles, and body. Cardio also makes your life easier and more enjoyable on a daily basis. Dynamic cardio sessions push your body beyond what is usually expected of it so that your daily activities become effortless. How is it going to feel when you walk up a flight of stairs and expend no more effort than when walking on level ground? I cannot emphasize enough that the body needs to operate as a calorie furnace. Become active in general; yearn for any event that raises your metabolism. Schedule your cardio workouts so that you never miss any. On days that you do miss your workout or you can't schedule time, boost your metabolism by using the stairs, taking a brisk walk between meetings, or performing other, similar activities. Then make sure that you get your exercise the next day. Tomorrow always offers a new start. Strive for excellence, not perfection.

"Those who think they have no time for bodily exercise will sooner or later have to find time for illness."

EDWARD STANLEY

Chapter Twenty-Seven

MUSCLE TONING

We have now arrived at the keystone of the *BetterBody BetterLife* program. I refer to it as a critical part because it is neglected by so many, and it is the difference between thin and fit. Muscle toning is the synergist. It makes 2 + 2 = 6 or 7 or even 8.

Don't lose weight. Lose *BODY FAT.*

Don't become thin. Become *FIT.*

Get healthy, toned, and fit. Diets alone certainly won't do it. Proper nutrition and cardiovascular exercise will do a good job, but to complete the harmony of the *Trilogy of Health*, you need to tone your muscles and make them stronger. A strong muscular structure will prevent injuries, increase mobility, increase metabolism, aid digestion, and assist your skeleton as it performs any activity you demand of it. By alternating between cardiovascular training and muscle toning and with the support of proper nutrition, you will create the body and life you have always dreamed about in less than 3 percent of your day.

DON'T GET THIN. GET FIT.

If you became twice as strong, would you feel half your weight? If you magnified that effect by losing body fat, you might feel three or four times lighter. Think of how nimble and buoyant you would feel. Just think how easy it would be to carry packages, move objects, get up from a chair, and move through life's travels. Muscle toning produces an exponential effect that allows you to become effortlessly active.

HOW MUSCLE TONING HELPS

- Aids in fat loss
- Increases metabolism
- Increases strength
- Tones your physique
- Fights obesity
- Slows the aging process
- Increases bone density, which fights osteoporosis
- Reduces risk of diabetes with increased glucose utilization
- Fights heart disease
- Reduces back pain
- Fights arthritis
- Improves athletic ability
- Promotes mental health (fights depression)
- Reduces cellulite*

*Cellulite cannot be spot eliminated; it must be reduced with the employment of a complete fitness plan. Reducing total body fat, eating right, toning muscles with resistance training, and conditioning with cardiovascular exercise are the only ways to reduce cellulite.

Resistance training strengthens and tones muscles. Resistance training is any activity that increases muscle strength. You have done some kind of resistance training although you may not be aware. Back in school, you probably did push-ups or pull-ups. As a child, you may have jumped rope or played piggyback with a friend. Even now you do resistance training every day – every time you pick up a package, sit down, stand up, open a door, or walk up stairs. As silly as it sounds, these activities are elementary level resistance training.

The most common forms of resistance training are calisthenics, yoga, power bands, universal gyms, circuit training, resistance equipment, and free-weight lifting. Although muscle-toning systems go by many names, all fit somewhere in one or more of those categories. A well-balanced fitness routine combines several and maybe even all of those techniques at one time or another. Every fitness model has muscle toning in his or her fitness plan. As a matter of fact, fitness models practice a lifestyle of proper nutrition, cardio training, and muscle toning to a precise degree.

To be most effective, resistance training needs to be performed at a dynamic level. Although such training means that you will be muscle toning with weights (or some other source of resistance), you will not train as a professional bodybuilder does.

Professional bodybuilders, like Mr. or Ms. Olympia, are at the extreme end of the spectrum. You will not train at the level of a professional, enduring a punishing cycle of lifting weights for hours each day. Professional athletes spend years of intense training and achieve pinpoint precision in diet and lifestyle to achieve their physiques. You won't go that far, so you will not bulk up to mammoth proportions.

Some women are afraid that they will get bulky when they start resistance training. If you are overfat and you start muscle toning, you might appear to be adding bulk, but you are not; your body is transforming. The appearance of bulk may result from a temporary increase in blood flow to the muscles when they are pumped during exercise. This temporary pump during exercise is what you are after. It means you are performing resistance training properly. With the application of the *Trilogy of Health* strategy (specifically proper nutrition and burning more calories than you consume), your body will tone and trim down, get rid of unwanted body fat, and leave you with a sleek, sexy, and trim physique that does not look muscular.

Female physiology makes building large and thick muscles difficult. Don't worry about building too much muscle; worry about not having enough. Creating a bulky, muscular, and massive body is a complex process, and it does not come easily. It requires years of highly intense and specific training. According to renowned strength-training researchers Steven J. Fleck and William J. Kraemer, the authors of *Designing Resistance Training Programs*, women typically don't gain size from strength training because, compared to men, they have ten to thirty times less of the hormones that cause bulking up.

In addition, muscle is dense and fat is bulky. One pound of body fat is many times larger than 1 pound of muscle. If you convert the same weight of body fat to muscle, the bulk will be as much as five times less. That means that your thighs, butt, arms, belly, and everything else will be considerably smaller. If you compound that effect with a reduction of body fat, then you will be left with a toned, fit, and incredible body.

CAN'T LOSE THE FAT?

As we age, the body loses muscle mass. Muscle burns more calories than body fat burns, and less muscle mass means a lower metabolism. That is, in part, why the body burns fewer calories as we age. Making this situation worse, improper dieting reduces muscle structure even more, making weight loss even more difficult. For those reasons, you must perform resistance training to tone and build muscles.

Without muscle toning to restore the muscle structure lost with age, weight-loss results are short-lived. Rebuilding and maintaining muscle structure is a keystone to weight loss and maintenance, as well as to a healthy life. Without muscle toning, the body continues its predisposition to weight gain; regaining lost weight — and adding more — are likely. A strong and toned body structure is the best way to lose fat and keep it off.

THE FURNACE

Every time you train your muscles, you burn calories and raise your metabolism. Your metabolism stays in this elevated state for several hours after the workout is over, so you burn many additional calories. When you add in proper nutrition, and cardiovascular conditioning, your body becomes a calorie-burning furnace. Muscle toning with resistance training completes the *Trilogy of Health* in creating a body that becomes and stays naturally lean.

TYPES OF RESISTANCE TRAINING

There are several ways to resistance train for muscle toning, and different people have different preferences. Calisthenics and yoga (the muscular aspects) are resistance training. They use the body's weight as resistance. Weights and machines take calisthenics to a higher level, but the principles are the same. Professional models and bodybuilders use calisthenics, free weights, and machine resistance training in their programs. Resistance training can be executed with multifunction universal gyms, resistance bands, free weights, and weight machines. Universal gyms are generally for the home fitness room. Circuit training and weight resistance machines are found in fitness clubs where the space and financial structure can support them. Free weights, free-weight machines, and universal machines can be found in the home and in the fitness club. New equipment is developed continually, and hybrids proliferate in the industry, often turning up as new fitness gadgets advertised on TV.

Many machines and exercises offer opportunities for strengthening your body and toning your muscles. Find the exercises that fit into your plan and use the facilities at your disposal. You can perform some variation of any exercise whether a machine is available to you or not. Simply choose the approach that works best for you given the facilities and equipment that you have.

I recommend a combination of styles for optimal results without boredom. I prefer using free weights as the staple for my resistance training. Free weights strengthen the targeted muscles and their stabilizing (supporting) muscles. Exercising complementary muscle groups promotes better balance and stability in real-life activities. For a nominal cost, you can have equipment at home. A few dumbbells in various sizes, an exercise bench, and a fitness band work great. I love fitness bands. They give a good, whole-body workout. Bands are portable and multifunctional. Bands take up almost no space and can easily fit into your briefcase or a suitcase when you travel. There is no reason to miss your routine when away from home. You may ultimately want more equipment, but fitness bands are a great place to start; and they should continue as a part of your exercise routine.

YOGA

I am frequently asked, "Is yoga considered strength training, and is it enough?" Yoga is a basic form of muscle strengthening and toning. It's wonderful for stretching and muscle endurance. However, it does not develop enough muscle strength to overcome the effects of age, nor does it force your muscles into growth for a strong and lean body. Yoga should be part of everyone's fitness program, but yoga is not enough.

QUALITY VERSUS QUANTITY

Quality of each repetition is important because of the exercise and rest cycle component to effective muscle toning. Quality repetitions reduce effort, while maximizing results. Careful, planned workouts and precise movements minimize the chance of injuries. Each muscle group needs to be conditioned with resistance training once a week. The rest of the week allows the muscles to recuperate. Muscles are stressed during each workout. The muscle membranes develop microscopic tears; they need time to repair. Your muscles become pumped during the training session; they repair and tone during rest. A haphazard workout creates unnecessary strain and damages your muscles. Adequate sleep is also important, especially when your body is going through a transformation.

BREATHE, BUT DON'T SWING

No, this isn't a new dance step. Perform each exercise using proper form and concentrating on the muscle being worked. Make each repetition slow and deliberate. Do not lower a weight quickly (on the negative), bounce, or cheat to lift the weight back; and do not swing your body during exercises. Cheating and body swinging reduce the effectiveness of the exercise and greatly increase the chance of injury. You may be lifting too heavy a weight if you're cheating or swinging the weight. From the starting position, lower the weight slowly while inhaling, pause for a second, and then lift the weight to the starting point while exhaling. Always exhale on the effort. Do not forget to breathe; breathing helps you keep the proper form and posture. Don't hold your breath. Holding your breath unnecessarily raises blood pressure.

TO GYM OR NOT TO GYM

Many people assume that to lose weight or to become toned and fit they need to join a local fitness club and work out all the time. Many believe that staying fit requires an athlete's lifestyle and hours at the fitness club; it does not. You can achieve exceptional results without joining a gym. You can become fit and stay lean in the comfort of your own home.

Some people feel embarrassed about exercising in a fitness club. They say, "Everyone will look at me and laugh at me." That isn't so. People in a fitness club generally come in all shapes and sizes. When you look around at them, you do not know who was once 50 pounds overweight. How do you think they got lean and fit? It wasn't from sitting on the couch wishing they were fit. Most people at the club are focused on their workout and not on others in the gym. Everyone in the gym is there to get or stay healthy.

HOME FITNESS CENTER OR FITNESS CLUB?

AT HOME

You can adopt a good fitness routine at home with a modest equipment budget, or you can have a fabulous home fitness center that will rival the local club. Which you choose depends on your budget, space, and willingness to commit a portion of your home to fitness. I wholeheartedly recommend a home gym to anyone who can afford one. On the other hand, if space or funds are at a premium, a local fitness club may be the best option.

I recommend home fitness centers for many reasons. Unless the local fitness club is close to home or close to work, you may make travel time your excuse for not exercising. At home, you can conveniently complete your fitness routine first thing in the morning. You can exercise, shower, and get ready for work, all in the comfort of your own home. Exercise can also be a way to unwind at the end of the workday, again in the privacy of your home. A home fitness center is, most likely, a must for full-time, at-home moms and dads. Working out at home requires no more time in your day then the 30 minutes it takes you to exercise. There is no travel time or down time. Home workouts also let you squeeze in fitness when other activities don't demand your attention, such as when the baby is napping. A home fitness center does have its drawbacks. You may have only a few pieces of equipment, and your interest may wane.

What you need at home: At a minimum, you should have a weight bench, a few dumbbells, a fitness band, and a small floor area. A multifunction gym bench that adjusts from a straight-up position to a flat position is useful. The bench allows you to perform presses, pull downs, back exercises, and more. Some benches can be used for leg curls, extensions, and squats. Other options are universal-type machines that have permanently installed weights. A different and newer version of this type of machine uses bows or bands as resistance.

AT THE FITNESS CLUB

Some people are not easily motivated to exercise at home, and some enjoy the atmosphere of a fitness club. The energy and bustle of the members working out in a fitness club can be inspirational. Fitness clubs usually offer classes as part of members' dues. Classes allow you to schedule exercise as you would an appointment. The advice and enthusiasm of a fitness instructor can be invaluable, too.

Joining a fitness club is an outstanding idea. At first, some people feel uncomfortable in a gym or health club. That's normal. Everyone feels a bit anxious in new surroundings. To overcome anxiety, go during off-peak hours or use the services of a personal trainer your first couple of times at the gym. A personal trainer's guided tour and demonstration of the equipment makes learning the exercises much easier. Many gyms offer two free sessions with a trainer when you join.

If you decide to employ a personal trainer on a long-term basis, try different people until you find a trainer who understands your goals and makes you feel comfortable. Take your *BetterBody BetterLife* plan to the fitness center and have your trainer show you how to implement the plan in his or her facility. Your trainer can show you the best machines and the best ways to accomplish your goals with that gym's facilities. Your initial consultation session should be free or inexpensive, or the cost may be applied to a package when you choose a trainer.

Warning: Today most clubs have up-to-date facilities, but some do not. I recommend a trial membership so you can preview a club and make sure it is right for you.

FITNESS CENTER MACHINES

Most fitness centers offer many machines you can choose from. More than one machine may exercise the same body part. Sometimes one machine isolates or emphasizes one part of the muscle, while another machine isolates a different part of the same muscle. For example, a chest press that uses a plane perpendicular to your torso tones the complete chest pectoral muscles. However, a chest press that has a plane of motion tilted toward your waist targets the lower pectoral muscles, while a plane of motion angled up toward your head targets your upper pectoral and frontal deltoid (shoulder) muscles. This same concept applies to inner and outer muscles in the arms, legs, and torso. Those who are working at beginning and intermediate levels should focus on exercises that work the entire muscle. Do not worry about getting fancy or complicated with your exercises. Keep your approach simple. Spend your energy on doing each exercise properly and intensely.

Gym etiquette requires all users of the facility to be considerate of others. All gyms will ask you to put equipment and weights back where they belong. At peak times, you may be limited to 20 or 30 minutes on cardiovascular equipment, or you may need to sign up for machines that are in high demand. You may need to use different pieces of equipment at peak times if you do not want to wait.

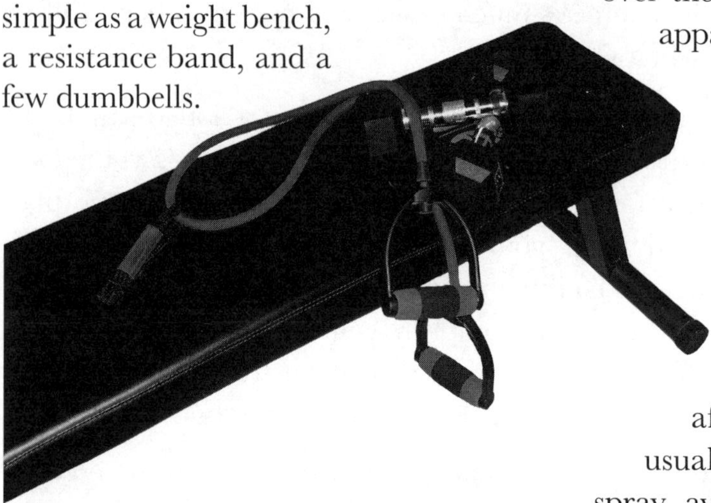

Home muscle toning equipment can be as simple as a weight bench, a resistance band, and a few dumbbells.

Often, people drape towels over the bench or pads of an apparatus while using that machine. If you have any skin contact with the equipment or if your clothes are damp from perspiring, wipe down the equipment after use. Good gyms usually have disinfectant spray available to clean the machines and the pads. If someone is resting between sets on resistance equipment and you need to use that equipment, simply ask to "work in." Most people will allow you to alternate turns on equipment with them.

FOR BEGINNERS

If you are a beginner to muscle toning and resistance training, the same rules apply as in cardiovascular conditioning. Make the first several weeks easy and light. Give your body time to learn the proper form and technique. I encourage you to use the help of a personal trainer or a fitness professional to teach your body the right way, the first time. Although most techniques are easy, all exercises require proper form to minimize the risk of injury and to maximize effectiveness. After the initial few weeks, you will begin to add resistance to gain strength and increase muscle toning.

> Note: You will not see toned muscles if you have a layer of body fat covering them. When you reduce your body fat percentage, you will see toned muscles, and when you continue to replace body fat with toned muscles, you will see a fit and toned physique.

IN THE SENIOR YEARS

The most important reason to have a strong and lean body is to improve physical performance and health. Do you remember 10 years ago how much easier it was to walk up a flight of stairs or to carry a bag of groceries? Wouldn't you like to have a strong and lean body again? As you age, your body degenerates if you do nothing to combat the effects of age and gravity. The older you grow, the harder recovery and rebuilding become. Still, it is never too late to start. Anyone can become as strong as he or she ever was, and maybe even stronger. At any age, especially in the senior years, a fit body makes the difference between being self-reliant and needing assistance to do common things. Fitness makes the difference between easily broken bones and a durable body. It is the difference between running with the pack and having everyone waiting for you to catch up. Imagine how great it will be when you can keep up with your children or grandchildren at Disneyland. You'll be an even better role model for your family and friends.

"Inward calm cannot be maintained unless physical strength is constantly and intelligently replenished."

**HINDU PRINCE GAUTAMA SIDDHARTA,
THE FOUNDER OF BUDDHISM**

Chapter Twenty-Eight

THE WORKOUT PLAN

The *BetterBody BetterLife* plan is designed with specific numbers of exercises, sets, repetitions, and rest periods to build strength, endurance, and toning. Exercising in this format maximizes results and minimizes effort. Throughout the workout, you will complete one set, rest 1 minute, and then do the next set. A 1-minute rest period between sets allows the muscles to recuperate sufficiently, but it is short enough to keep the muscles in a proper state for toning and strengthening.

Each body part needs to be worked to fatigue, which means you will perform the exercise (excluding warmup) until you cannot lift or repeat the motion again. For each exercise, you need to determine how much weight, or resistance, allows you to perform the desired number of repetitions (reps). For most exercises, you will do 12 reps for each set. That number develops endurance, while strengthening and toning your physique. When you get to the last rep, you should not be able to do another, and your muscles should burn. The burn is a temporary sensation that you feel when your muscles are stressed. If you can do more than 12 reps, then increase the weight. If you can't reach 12 reps, then reduce the weight appropriately. The idea is to force the muscle to become stronger without injuring yourself.

When performing strength training to fatigue with free weights, a spotter can help you, if needed. A partner (or spotter) provides motivation, keeps watch, and gives slight assistance as you reach the point of fatigue if you are unable to complete a set on your own. You and your partner can take turns spotting for each other. Many machines do not require a spotter for safe, solo operation. Check the machine's instructions.

Notice that the first exercise of the day is completed at 50 percent of your maximum resistance or weightlifting capacity. The next set is completed at 80 percent; and the third, at 100 percent for 12 repetitions. After these first sets, your muscles will be prewarmed so you won't need to start the subsequent sets at the warmup level. When you move on to the next body part, the first set can safely be performed at 100 percent of your maximum weightlifting ability, again for 12 repetitions.

For example, after you have done the three sets of chest presses to target your pectoral muscles, your triceps, biceps (arms), and deltoids (shoulders) are warmed from their supporting role in the exercise. A chest press targets your pectoral muscles specifically, but not exclusively. The other muscles work as supporting muscles or secondary muscles to the exercise. Consequently, they are warmed up. The plan is designed to take advantage of this effect. Each day, the starting exercises will warm up the other muscles that will be trained in the following sets. Therefore, subsequent muscles in the same muscle group will not need the warmup sets.

THE WORKOUT SCHEDULE

The first day of a new week offers the opportunity to start fresh. If you missed a workout, then this is the week to resolve to miss none and to move closer to your goals. Everyone misses workouts occasionally. Each day or each week is a new chance to get it right. Never stop trying!

Don't strive for perfection. Strive for progress.

YOUR WEEK AT A GLANCE

Muscle Toning — Monday, Wednesday, Friday
Cardiovascular Conditioning — Tuesday, Thursday, Saturday

° Monday °

30-minute muscle toning – ***Upper body*** (chest, shoulders and arms)

° Tuesday °

30-minute cardio – Stair climber*

° Wednesday °

30-minute muscle toning – ***Legs*** (quadriceps, hamstrings, calves)

° Thursday °

30-minute cardio – Stationary bicycle*

° Friday °

30-minute muscle toning – ***Back and Abs*** (back, latissimus, and abs)

° Saturday °

30-minute cardio – Treadmill*

° Sunday °

Day off

*Choose any cardio that you enjoy.
(See Cardiovascular Conditioning Section)

Sunday - Active Day Off

Sunday is your day off. Don't plan exercise or a dynamic workout for that day. It is your day to recoup and rejuvenate. You may find that you won't want to take the day off, and you will do something positive for your body or life. Listen to your conscience and use every day effectively.

Although this is a rest day, it should be a day of active rest. You will rest from your workout but not from being active. Run errands, go to the beach, or to take the kids to the park. Taking it easy is good, and your body needs time to recuperate, but "vegging out" all day on the couch will only make you look like a potato.

Variations to Work into Your Lifestyle

Cardio:

Activity:	Replace with:
Stair climber	Walking briskly (jogging) though the neighborhood
	Walking up and down the stairs in your building
	Dancing
	Hiking

Stationary Bicycle	Bicycling through the park
	Paddleboating in the park
	Swimming laps at the town pool or lake
Treadmill	Walking briskly (jogging) with your dog
	Walking to the train station or work
	Rollerblading or rollerskating

MUSCLE TONING:

Leg Presses	Hiking (mountains, steep grade)
	Cutting the lawn (push mower)
Upper Body	Working in the yard
	Rock climbing
	Playing most sports
	Doing yoga

Investing 30 minutes a day will get you into the best shape of your life. Everyone can find or make 30 minutes in a day. If you say, "I'm so busy, there is no way I can fit in a half hour a day to work out," then you're looking for an excuse to stay the way you are. There is no magic pill or elixir that can change your body and your life. You need to take the first step. In a short time, you will make up for the 30 minutes a day. You will get more done in less time, your mind will be clearer, you will perform more efficiently, and you will see the doctor a lot less often. A friend reported to me, "Since I lost 36 pounds I feel lighter! Really, I FEEL lighter!" Then he jumped in the air with a big smile and a giggle, as if someone were lifting him. He went on to reach his goal and lost another 22 pounds. This is a small commitment to change your life. Wouldn't you love to feel lighter? Give yourself a half hour a day, and you will have a ***better body*** and a ***better life***.

Life is short. Make it fun. Make it worthwhile.

MONDAY

1 Chest
Pectoral Muscles (pecs) 5 sets

- 1st Set – Chest Press
50% max weight 20 Reps (warmup)
Rest 1 minute
- 2nd Set – Chest Press
80% of max weight for 12 reps
Rest 1 minute
- 3rd Set – Chest Press
100% of max weight for 12 reps
Rest 1 minute
- 4th Set – Pec Flyes
100% of max weight for 12 reps
Rest 1 minute
- 5th Set – Pec Flyes
100% of max weight for 12 reps
Rest 1 minute

2 Shoulders
Deltoids – 4 Sets

- 1st Set – Shoulder Press
100% of max weight for 12 Reps
Rest 1 minute
- 2nd Set – Shoulder Press
100% of max weight for 12 reps
Rest 1 minute
- 3rd Set – Lateral Raises
100% of max weight for 12 reps
Rest 1 minute
- 4th Set – Lateral Raises
100% of max weight for 12 reps
Rest 1 minute

3 Biceps
Front of upper arm – 3 Sets

- 1st Set – Dumbbell Curls
100 % of max weight for 12 Reps
Rest 1 minute
- 2nd Set – Dumbbell Curls
100% of max weight for 12 reps
Rest 1 minute
- 3rd Set – Dumbbell Curls
100% of max weight for 12 reps

4 Triceps
Back of upper arm – 3 Sets

- 1st Set – Tri Extensions
100 % of max weight for 12 Reps
Rest 1 minute
- 2nd Set – Tri Extensions
100% of max weight for 12 reps
Rest 1 minute
- 3rd Set – Triceps Pull-Downs
100% of max weight for 12 reps

Monday workout completed – Stretch all muscles

TUESDAY

Cardio Day (see page 168)

3-minute warmup
20 minutes of dynamic cardiovascular conditioning
2 minutes of cool down
5 minutes of stretching

WEDNESDAY

1 Quadriceps (Quads)
Front of upper leg – 7 Sets

- 1st Set – Dumbbell Squats

50% max weight 20 Reps (warmup)
Rest 1 minute

- 2nd Set – Dumbbell Squats

80% of max weight for 12 reps
Rest 1 minute

- 3rd Set – Dumbbell Squats

100% of max weight for 12 reps
Rest 1 minute

- 4th Set – Dumbbell Squats

100% of max weight for 12 reps
Rest 1 minute

- 5th Set – Leg Extensions

100% of max weight for 12 reps
Rest 1 minute

- 6th Set – Leg Extensions

100% of max weight for 12 reps
Rest 1 minute

- 7th Set – Leg Extensions

100% of max weight for 12 reps
Rest 1 minute

3 Calves
Back of lower leg – 3 Sets

- 1st Set – Calf Raises

100% of max weight for 12 Reps
Rest 1 minute

- 2nd Set – Calf Raises

100% of max weight for 12 reps
Rest 1 minute

- 3rd Set – Calf Raises

100% of max weight for 12 reps
Rest 1 minute

2 Hamstrings
Back of upper leg – 5 Sets

- 1st Set – Lunges

100% of max weight for 12 reps
Rest 1 minute

- 2nd Set – Lunges

100% of max weight for 12 reps
Rest 1 minute

- 3rd Set – Lunges

100% of max weight for 12 reps
Rest 1 minute

- 4th Set – Leg Curl

100% of max weight for 12 reps
Rest 1 minute

- 5th Set – Leg Curl

100% of max weight for 12 reps
Rest 1 minute

Wednesday workout complete
Stretch all muscles

THURSDAY

Cardio Day (See page 168)
3-minute warmup
20 minutes of dynamic
cardiovascular conditioning
2 minutes of cool down
5 minutes of stretching

FRIDAY

1 Latissimus Dorsi (Lats)
Wing-shaped muscles under arms

• 1st Set – Lat Pull-Downs
20 Reps (warm up set)
Start with 50% of max weight
Rest 1 minute

• 2nd Set – Lat Pull-Downs
100% of max weight for 12 reps
Rest 1 minute

• 3rd Set – Lat Pull-Downs
100% of max weight for 12 reps
Rest 1 minute

• 4th Set – Close Grip Pull-Downs
100% of max weight for 12 reps
Rest 1 minute

• 5th Set – Close Grip Pull-Downs
100% of max weight for 12 reps
Rest 1 minute

3 Abdominal (Abs)
Stomach/torso muscles
"The Six Pack" – 5 Sets

• 1st Set – Leg Lifts
12 Reps - Rest 1 minute

• 2nd Set – Leg Lifts
12 Reps - Rest 1 minute

• 3rd Set – Crunches
12 Reps - Rest 1 minute

• 4th Set – Crunches
12 Reps - Rest 1 minute

• 5th Set – Crunches
12 Reps - Rest 1 minute

2 *BACK*
5 Sets

• 1st Set – Rows
12 Reps (warm up set)
Start with 80% of maximum weight
Rest 1 minute

• 2nd Set – Rows
100% of max weight for 12 reps
Rest 1 minute

• 3rd Set – Rows
100% of max weight for 12 reps
Rest 1 minute

• 4th Set – One-Arm Dumbbell Rows (each arm)
100% of max weight for 12 reps
Rest 1 minute

• 5th Set – One-Arm Dumbbell Rows (each arm)
100% of max weight for 12 reps
Rest 1 minute

Friday workout complete
Stretch all muscles

SATURDAY

Cardio Day (See page 168)
3-minute warmup
20 minutes of dynamic cardiovascular conditioning
2 minutes of cool down
5 minutes of stretching

Chapter Twenty-Nine

THE JOURNAL

The journal brings the whole *BetterBody BetterLife* program together. Without a journal, you stand little chance of judging and improving your progress. Studies show that using a journal to record goals, plans, and progress and to review the journey helps individuals achieve greater success in any goal. Your journal will coach you and make fitness management easier. Follow the steps, plan your days, and record everything so you can build on your strengths and diminish your weaknesses.

In the following pages, you will find a week of the *BetterBody BetterLife Fitness Journal*. The journal is a simple format that is easy to use, update, and apply consistently.

The journal offers a two-page spread for each day. The left-hand pages are nutrition pages to use for planning and recording everything that you eat or drink. In the left columns of the nutrition pages, plan your meals and midmeals for the day, including your fluids. You can plan in the morning, the night before, or even a week in advance. Throughout the day, record in the columns on the right everything that you actually consume: meals, snacks, midmeals, soft drinks, and even water.

At the bottom of the page, write some notes about your day; include successes, weaknesses, emotions, and improvement ideas. Recording everything that you consume and your emotions when you eat will help you determine your eating habits, patterns, strengths, and weaknesses. Many people are surprised by some of the food choices they make or how much food they consume unwittingly.

The right-hand pages of the *BetterBody BetterLife Journal* are the exercise pages. As you did for nutrition, fill in your plan for muscle toning or cardiovascular conditioning in the columns on the left and your actual workout on the right. On muscle toning days, if you are doing the same exercises that are already entered in gray, then you do nothing with those spaces. However, those exercises are only recommendations; if you want or need to make a change, write over the gray writing. In the right columns, fill in the actual exercises you performed, the number of repetitions, and the quality of the effort you put into each exercise expressed as a percentage of your ability.

On the cardio days, the journal works in the same way. Fill in your planned exercise, the time you will start, and the number of minutes. Then in the horizontal boxes, fill in your actual level of intensity. Make some notes on these pages, too.

In the top right-hand corner of the nutrition pages, you will find "______ STARS" for rating your day. In that space, fill in your overall assessment of the day on a scale from 1 (needs a lot of improvement) to 10 (an outstanding day). To do this, consider how well you planned and followed your nutrition, how well you exercised, and how your day went in general. Did you plan effectively? Were you more active throughout the day? Did you drink four bottles of water? Did you exercise or do muscle toning? Did you give your workout an all-out effort or were you just going through the motions? After considering everything, rate your day from 1 to 10. Nobody is perfect, but your average should be 7 and above. A rating of 7 means that you followed your plan and exercised, but you still have a little room for improvement. A rating of 6 or below means you missed something significant, such as planning, exercising, or eating nutritiously.

DAY SEVEN

Day seven is your day off. Although you have one day a week where you are not dynamically exercising, your "day off" is still a factor in your overall health plan. A day off does not mean you can be a couch potato for 16 hours! This is an active rest day, meaning that you should be doing things with your family, working in the yard, running errands, or playing sports. Maybe day seven is the crazy day at work where you cannot find the time to work out. You are still eating well on day seven, right? That said, sometimes your body needs a day or a half-day for rest. The body is not a machine. It will give you signals and signs when you should take things easy. If your body is talking to you, listen! Rest and recover to avoid injury.

It is the end of the week. - So, how did you do?

Did you plan your days?

Did you follow your plan every day or most days?

Did you eat quality foods each day?

Did you do muscle toning three days?

Did you do cardio exercise three days?

Did you fill in your journal and assess your efforts?

What did you do great?

What do you need to improve?

What can you do to improve?

The last two pages of each week provide space for reviewing and evaluating how you did during the past week. What was your biggest successes, and what were your biggest obstacles?

On the top of the left-hand page, write about what you did best that week. Give yourself some accolades. Write about your successes and breakthroughs. Include only positive back-patting in this part. Write about everything that you did well. Note your best nutrition days and your best exercise days. What was great about your cardio workouts and your muscle-toning workouts? Where did you make your biggest breakthroughs?

The lower part of the left-hand page provides space so you can write about what you need to improve. Discuss your weaknesses and greatest obstacles. What aspect of your nutrition plan needs a change for the better? Did you exercise every day? Did you do all three cardio workouts and all three muscle-toning workouts?

On the right-hand page, write about the lessons you learned during that week. Figure out how you can improve. For example, "I missed my Monday workout because I was running late. Next week I will make sure I get to bed on time the night before so that I do not hit the snooze button three times. I will get up on time so that I do not miss my workout again." This section should be positive and uplifting, but honest. You did not fail if you learned from your past actions. On this page, write about how you feel and how you grew as a person during the past week. If you do not feel good or great about the past week, then write about why and how you can improve. Spending a few minutes during your off day to reflect on your past efforts and find ways to improve is always a good investment of time. Your weekly review will also help you get motivated and focused for the coming week.

And finally fill in your stars. The rating is from 1 to 10 stars.

How many stars this week?
Overall, your week?
Overall, meals and nutrition?
Powerfests?
Lunches?
Dinners?
Midmeals?
Cardio workouts?
Muscle-toning workouts?
How do you feel?
What is your current weight?
Did you lose weight (or maintain)?
Did you have a 10-star week?

A journal is an exceptional way to plan, record progress, and savor some thoughts. Much of what you record settles into your subconscious. There it becomes an integral part of you. Journals are insightful, rewarding, and — if used consistently — highly effective in helping you reach your goals. Strive for progress, not perfection. Missing a goal is not failure; failure is not moving closer to your goal.

"Journal writing is a voyage to the interior."

CHRISTINA BALDWIN

ON THE FOLLOWING 14 PAGES:
A WEEK OF JOURNAL PAGES

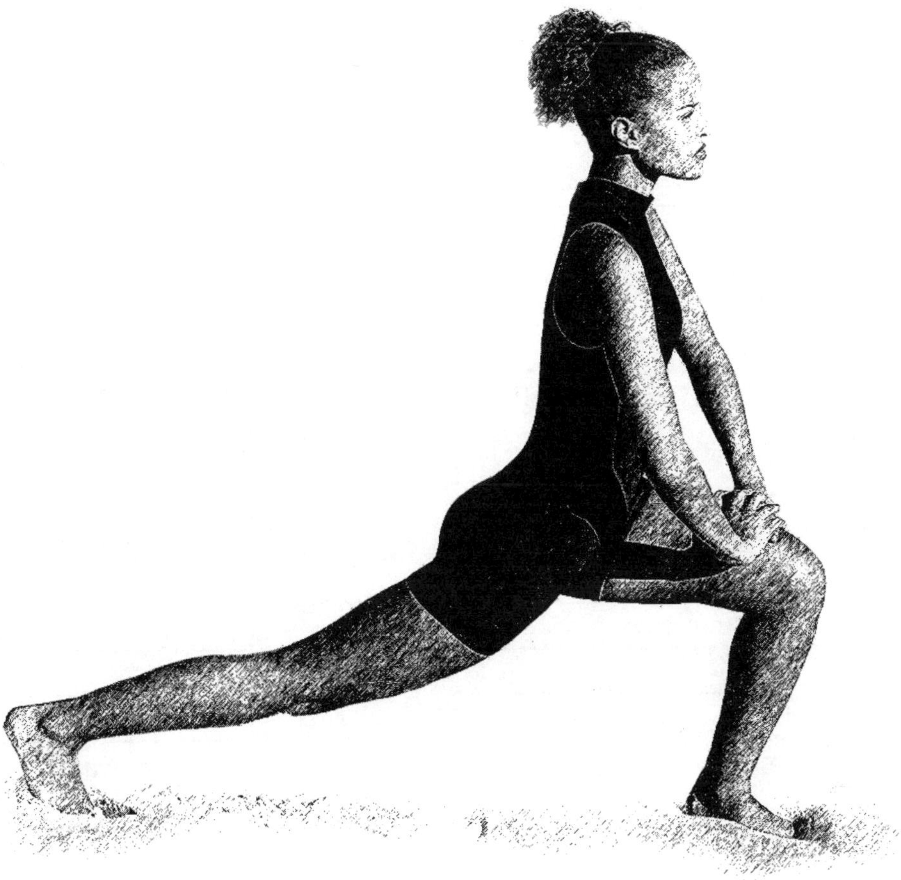

NUTRITION

DAY 1 (MONDAY) ____________________ ____________ STARS

Week ________ Date ______________ Rate the day (1-10) Nutrition & exercise

Planned Nutrition			Actual Nutrition
Powerfest Time		**Powerfest** Time	
Midmeal Time		**Midmeal** Time	
Lunch Time		**Lunch** Time	
Midmeal Time		**Midmeal** Time	
Dinner Time		**Dinner** Time	
	Bottles of water 4		Bottles of water ______

Notes:

MUSCLE TONING

UPPER BODY - Chest, Shoulders, & Arms

Planned Start Time ____________ Actual Start Time ____________

Planned Exercise			
Exercise	Reps	Resistance	Minutes Rest
CHEST			
Chest Press	20	50%	1
Chest Press	12	80%	1
Chest Press	12	100%	1
Pec Flyes	12	100%	1
Pec Flyes	12	100%	1
SHOULDERS			
Shoulder Press	12	100%	1
Shoulder Press	12	100%	1
Lateral Raises	12	100%	1
Lateral Raises	12	100%	1
BICEPS			
Dumbbell Curls	12	100%	1
Dumbbell Curls	12	100%	1
Dumbbell Curls	12	100%	1
TRICEPS			
Tri Extensions	12	100%	1
Tri Extensions	12	100%	1
Tri Pull-Downs	12	100%	1

Actual Exercise			
Exercise	Reps	Resistance	Minutes Rest
CHEST			
SHOULDERS			
BICEPS			
TRICEPS			

Note: Exercises filled in gray are suggested. Fill in the exercise that you choose to do.

Note: Resistance column is the weight used or the resistance number.

Notes:

NUTRITION

DAY 2 (TUESDAY) ____________________ ____________ STARS

Week ________ Date ________________ Rate the day (1-10) Nutrition & exercise

Planned Nutrition		Actual Nutrition	
Powerfest Time ____		**Powerfest** Time ____	
Midmeal Time ____		**Midmeal** Time ____	
Lunch Time ____		**Lunch** Time ____	
Midmeal Time ____		**Midmeal** Time ____	
Dinner Time ____		**Dinner** Time ____	
Bottles of water 4		Bottles of water ____	

Notes:

CARDIOVASCULAR EXERCISE

30-Minute Cardio Workout

Planned Start Time ____________ Actual Start Time____________

Planned Minutes Exercised ______ Actual Minutes Exercised ______

Planned Exercise	Actual Exercise
____________________	____________________

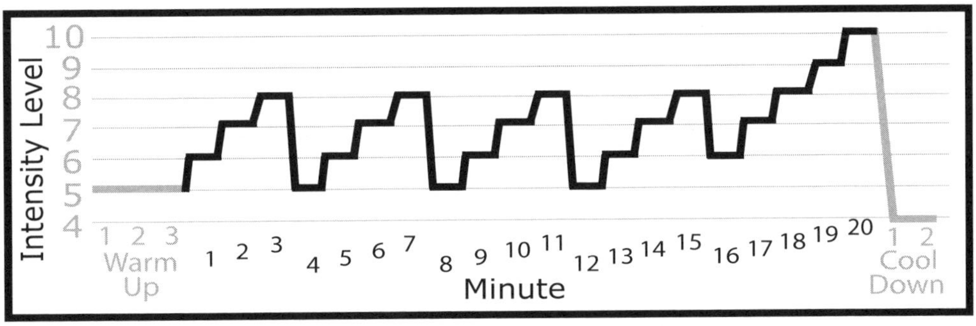

Minute	Warm Up			1	2	3	4	5	6	7	8	9	10
Planned Intensity	5	5	5	6	7	8	5	6	7	8	5	6	7
Actual Intensity													

Minute	11	12	13	14	15	16	17	18	19	20	Cool Down	
Planned Intensity	8	5	6	7	8	6	7	8	9	10	4	4
Actual Intensity												

Always warm up, cool down, and stretch after exercising

Notes:

JOURNAL

NUTRITION

DAY 3 (WEDNESDAY)________________ ________ STARS

Week ________ Date ____________ Rate the day (1-10) Nutrition & exercise

Planned Nutrition		Actual Nutrition	
Powerfest Time		**Powerfest** Time	
Midmeal Time		**Midmeal** Time	
Lunch Time		**Lunch** Time	
Midmeal Time		**Midmeal** Time	
Dinner Time		**Dinner** Time	
Bottles of water 4		Bottles of water ____	

Notes:

MUSCLE TONING

LEGS - Quads, Hamstrings & Calves

Planned Start Time______________ Actual Start Time______________

Planned Exercise				Actual Exercise			
Exercise	Reps	Resistance	Minutes Rest	Exercise	Reps	Resistance	Minutes Rest
QUADS							
Squats	20	50%	1				
Squats	12	80%	1				
Squats	12	100%	1				
Squats	12	100%	1				
Leg Extensions	12	100%	1				
Leg Extensions	12	100%	1				
Leg Extensions	12	100%	1				
HAMSTRINGS							
Lunges	12	100%	1				
Lunges	12	100%	1				
Lunges	12	100%	1				
Leg Curls	12	100%	1				
Leg Curls	12	100%	1				
CALVES							
Calf Raises	12	100%	1				
Calf Raises	12	100%	1				
Calf Raises	12	100%	1				

Note: Exercises filled in gray are suggested. Fill in the exercise that you choose to do.

Note: Resistance column is the weight used or the resistance number.

Notes:

NUTRITION

DAY 4 (THURSDAY) ________________ ________ STARS

Week ________ Date ______________ Rate the day (1-10) Nutrition & exercise

	Planned Nutrition		**Actual Nutrition**
Powerfest Time ____		**Powerfest** Time ____	
Midmeal Time ____		**Midmeal** Time ____	
Lunch Time ____		**Lunch** Time ____	
Midmeal Time ____		**Midmeal** Time ____	
Dinner Time ____		**Dinner** Time ____	
	Bottles of water 4		Bottles of water ____

Notes:

CARDIOVASCULAR EXERCISE

30-Minute Cardio Workout

Planned Start Time ____________ Actual Start Time____________

Planned Minutes Exercised ______ Actual Minutes Exercised ______

Planned Exercise

____

Actual Exercise

____

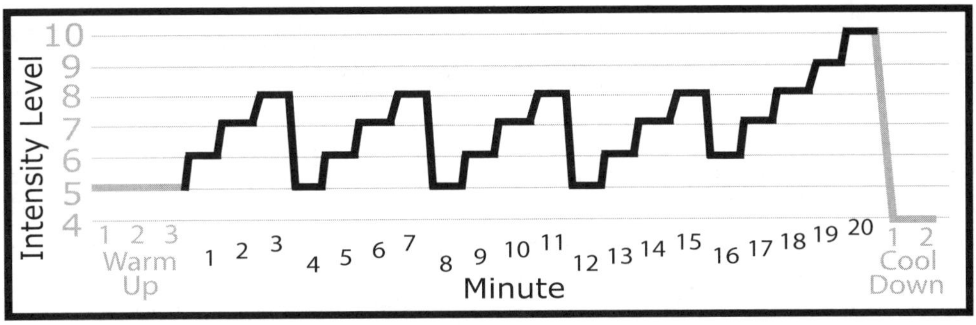

Minute	Warm Up			1	2	3	4	5	6	7	8	9	10
Planned Intensity	5	5	5	6	7	8	5	6	7	8	5	6	7
Actual Intensity													

Minute	11	12	13	14	15	16	17	18	19	20	Cool Down	
Planned Intensity	8	5	6	7	8	6	7	8	9	10	4	4
Actual Intensity												

Always warm up, cool down, and stretch after exercising

Notes:

NUTRITION

DAY 5 (FRIDAY) ____________________ ____________ STARS

Week ________ Date ________________ Rate the day (1-10) Nutrition & exercise

Planned Nutrition		Actual Nutrition	
Powerfest Time ____		**Powerfest** Time ____	
Midmeal Time ____		**Midmeal** Time ____	
Lunch Time ____		**Lunch** Time ____	
Midmeal Time ____		**Midmeal** Time ____	
Dinner Time ____		**Dinner** Time ____	
Bottles of water 4		Bottles of water ____	

Notes:

MUSCLE TONING

UPPER BODY - Back, Lats, & Abs

Planned Start Time______________ Actual Start Time______________

Planned Exercise				Actual Exercise			
Exercise	Reps	Resistance	Minutes Rest	Exercise	Reps	Resistance	Minutes Rest
LATS							
Lat Pull Down	20	50%	1				
Lat Pull Down	12	80%	1				
Lat Pull Down	12	100%	1				
Close Grip Pull Dn	12	100%	1				
Close Grip Pull Dn	12	100%	1				
BACK							
Rows	12	80%	1				
Rows	12	100%	1				
Rows	12	100%	1				
One Arm-Rows	12	100%	1				
One Arm-Rows	12	100%	1				
ABS							
Leg Lifts	12	-	1				
Leg Lifts	12	-	1				
Crunches	12	-	1				
Crunches	12	-	1				
Crunches	12	-	1				

Note: Exercises filled in gray are suggested. Fill in the exercise that you choose to do.

Note: Resistance column is the weight used or the resistance number.

Notes:

NUTRITION

DAY 6 (SATURDAY) ________________

Week ________ Date ______________

__________ STARS
Rate the day (1-10)
Nutrition & exercise

Planned Nutrition		Actual Nutrition	
Powerfest Time		**Powerfest** Time	
Midmeal Time		**Midmeal** Time	
Lunch Time		**Lunch** Time	
Midmeal Time		**Midmeal** Time	
Dinner Time		**Dinner** Time	
Bottles of water	4	Bottles of water	

Notes:

CARDIOVASCULAR EXERCISE

30-Minute Cardio Workout

Planned Start Time ____________ Actual Start Time ____________

Planned Minutes Exercised ______ Actual Minutes Exercised ______

Planned Exercise	Actual Exercise
____________________	____________________

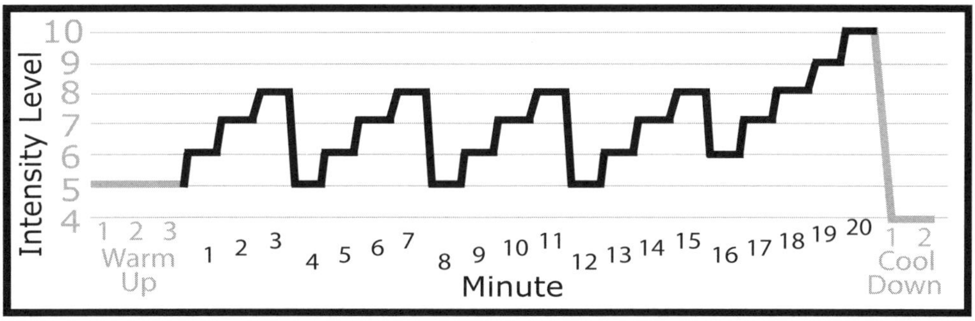

Minute	Warm Up			1	2	3	4	5	6	7	8	9	10
Planned Intensity	5	5	5	6	7	8	5	6	7	8	5	6	7
Actual Intensity													

Minute	11	12	13	14	15	16	17	18	19	20	Cool Down	
Planned Intensity	8	5	6	7	8	6	7	8	9	10	4	4
Actual Intensity												

Always warm up, cool down, and stretch after exercising

Notes:

JOURNAL

DAY 7 (SUNDAY) ______________

Week ______ Date ______________

Week in Review

ACCOLADES (Write about the positive events of the week. Back-patting only.)

Notes:

NEEDS IMPROVEMENT (Write about your weaknesses needing improvement.)

Notes:

JOURNAL

STARS 1 - 10		WEEK OVERALL	STARS 1 - 10	
Powerfests	______		______	Cardio Workouts
Lunches	______	___	______	Muscle Toning
Dinners	______	STARS	______	Daily Activity
Midmeals	______		______	How You Feel

Your Current Weight ________

Loss / Gain ________

Notes: (Lessons learned)

BODY PART	EXERCISE OPTIONS	
CHEST	Barbell bench press Dumbbell bench press Incline bench press	Dumbbell flyes Machine flyes (pec deck) Cable crossovers (flyes)
SHOULDERS	Barbell press Dumbbell press	Lateral raises Frontal raises
BICEPS	Barbell curls Dumbbell curls Preacher curls	Cable curls Machine curls Seated dumbbell curls
TRICEPS	Barbell tricep extensions One-arm tricep extensions Cable press down	Tricep dips Tricep presses Dumbbell kickbacks
LATS	Close-grip pull-down Wide-grip pull-down	Close-grip chin-up Wide-grip chin-up
BACK	Bent over dumbbell rows Bent over barbell rows	Cable rows One-arm rows
ABS	Crunches Abdominal curls Machine curls	Lying leg raises Hanging leg raises Knee raises
QUADS	Dumbbell squats Barbell squats	Leg extensions Machine leg presses
HAM-STRINGS	Lunges Leg curls	Straight-leg deadlifts
CALVES	Standing calf raises Seated calf raises	Machine calf raises Donkey calf raises

Some exercise options require specialized equipment found in a fitness club. Please seek a personal trainer for assistance.

Chapter Thirty

THE EXERCISE GUIDE

To help you get a quick start, I have included the *BetterBody BetterLife Muscle Toning* video DVD with your program. Proper form is very important to maximize results and minimize risks. Photographs are not the best way to teach proper form, and photographs of instructions won't motivate you. For those reasons, I created the DVD.

The video provides a step-by-step guide with my commentary and instructions on how to do the muscle-toning exercises. It also shows some alternate ways to accomplish the same moves. For example, you can do bicep curls with a fitness band or with free weights. The way you work out at home is likely to be different from the way that you work out at a fitness club.

The exercises are shown in the same order as the exercise plan. Perform each exercise slowly and accurately. Fast movements and cheating to perform the exercise will increase your chances of injury and cheat you out of the full benefits of the workout. If you have any questions in performing any exercise, please consult a certified personal trainer or other qualified instructor. Safety is always the first priority.

This program is designed to work on all major muscle groups. Follow the instructions in the video. In a short time, you will comfortably remember and perform all of the exercises.

Be safe and have fun.
Remember, it's all about attitude.

"The only way to predict the future is to create it."

Chapter Thirty-One

DREAM IT, PLAN IT, DO IT

As a great friend of mine tells me, "Dream it! Plan it! Do it!" You have the dream. You purchased this book so you can plan for your dream. Now you must achieve your dream. Move toward your goals every day, and you will succeed. You now have the knowledge to complete any fitness goal you have set. Look forward and you will move forward. Do not neglect or forget to appreciate each accomplishment and gift in your life, for each day is a treasure. Give life your best.

Live fit. Work hard. Play harder. Laugh often. Love most!

Life is a wonderful ride!

Warmest wishes,

Croix

Dream It, Plan It, Do It

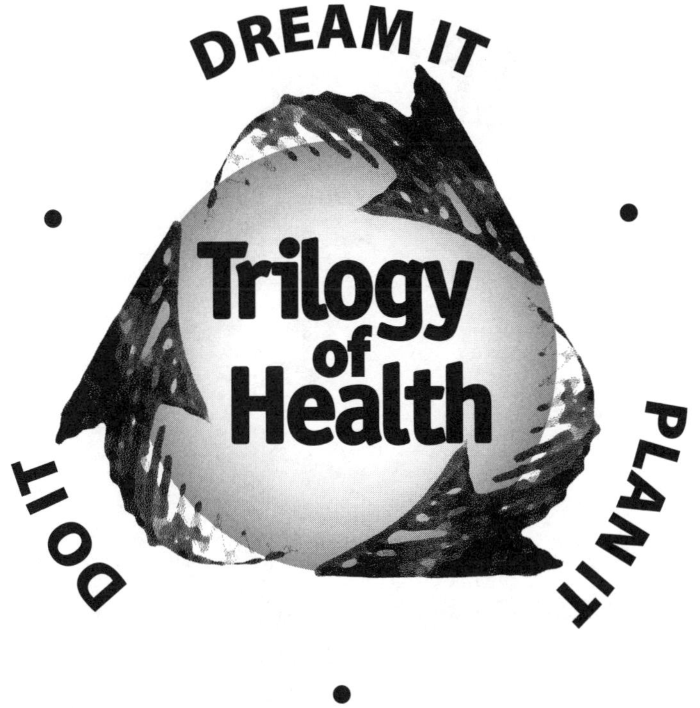

"If you always do what you have always done,

You will always get what you always got!"

APPENDIX

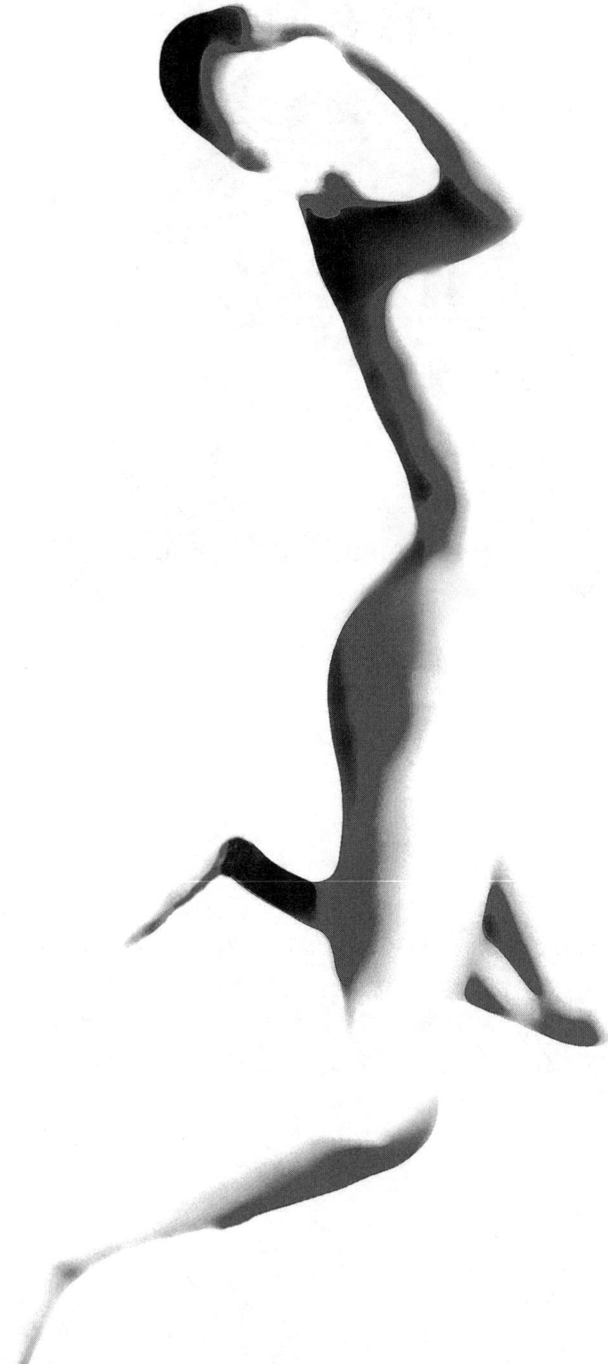

MY STARTING POINT

NAME	
DATE	
AGE	
WEIGHT	
HEIGHT	
BMI	

MEASUREMENTS

WAIST	
HIPS	
CHEST	
THIGHS	
ARMS	
PANT SIZE	

DREAMS TO GOALS

BMI
BODY MASS INDEX CHART

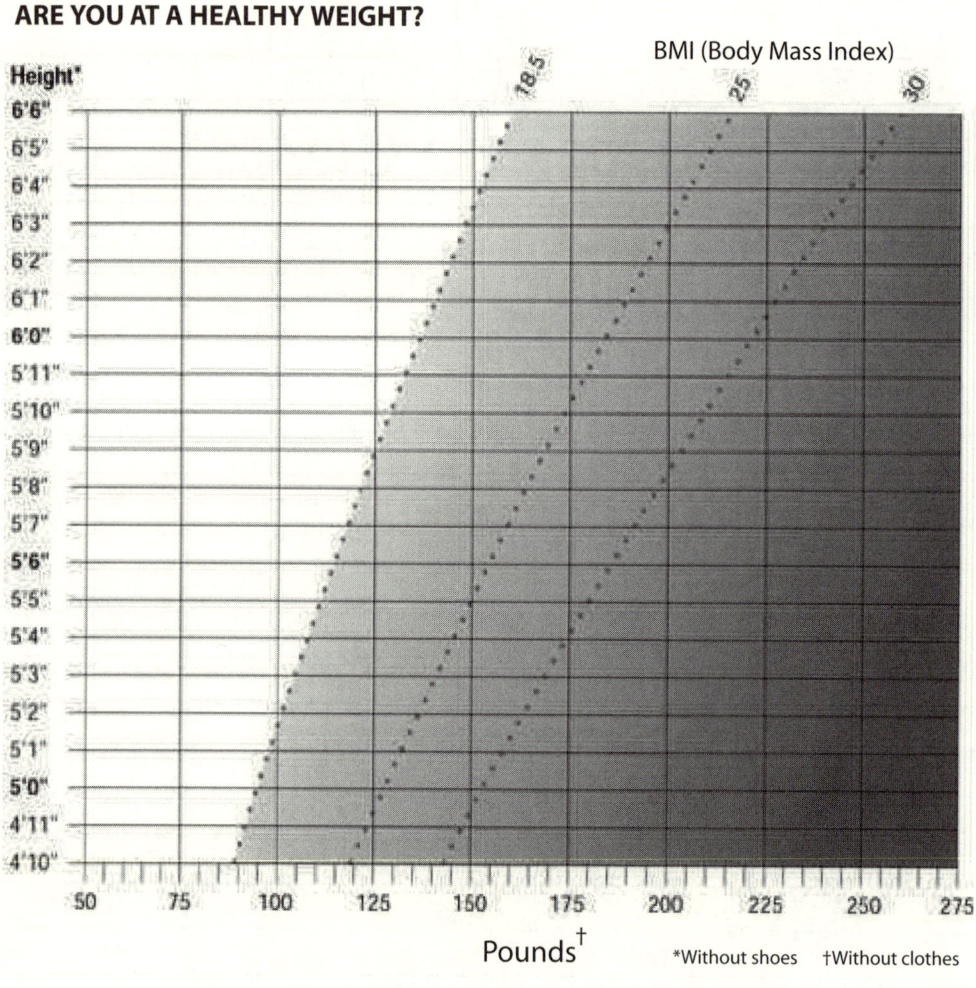

Reprinted from the U.S. Food and Drug Administration

The U.S. FDA Body Mass Index is a guideline. Your frame, structure and gender must be considered when determining if you are of a healthy weight or unhealthy weight. A better indication is your body fat percentage, your physique, your physical fitness, how you feel, and how you look in the mirror.

HEART RATE

MAXIMUM HEART RATE
220 - your age

TARGET HEART RATE ZONE
80% of your maximum HR

Note: Some medical conditions may lower the maximum heart rate and thus the target zone rate. Consult your physician to find out if you need to use a lower target heart rate.

YOUR WEEK AT A GLANCE

Muscle Toning — Monday, Wednesday, Friday
Cardiovascular Conditioning — Tuesday, Thursday, Saturday

° MONDAY °
30-minute muscle toning – ***Upper body*** (chest, shoulders and arms)

° TUESDAY °
30-minute cardio – Stair climber*

° WEDNESDAY °
30-minute muscle toning – ***Legs*** (quadriceps, hamstrings, calves)

° THURSDAY °
30-minute cardio – Stationary bicycle*

° FRIDAY °
30-minute muscle toning – ***Back and Abs*** (back, latissimus, and abs)

° SATURDAY °
30-minute cardio – Treadmill*

° SUNDAY °
Day off

*Choose any cardio that you enjoy.
(See Cardiovascular Conditioning Section)

MUSCLE CHART

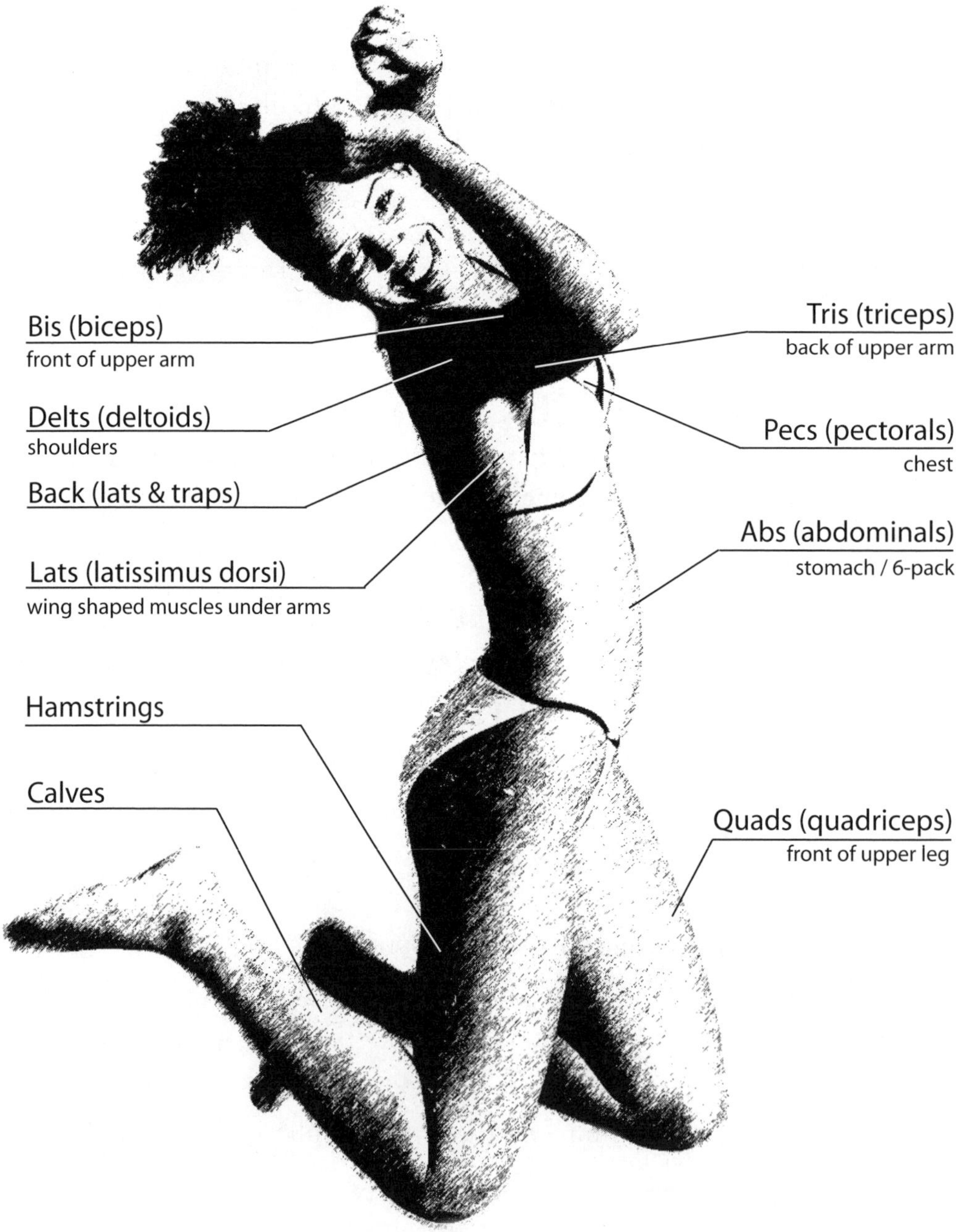

APPENDIX

BODY PART	EXERCISE OPTIONS	
CHEST	Barbell bench press Dumbbell bench press Incline bench press	Dumbbell flyes Machine flyes (pec deck) Cable crossovers (flyes)
SHOULDERS	Barbell press Dumbbell press	Lateral raises Frontal raises
BICEPS	Barbell curls Dumbbell curls Preacher curls	Cable curls Machine curls Seated dumbbell curls
TRICEPS	Barbell tricep extensions One-arm tricep extensions Cable press down	Tricep dips Tricep presses Dumbbell kickbacks
LATS	Close-grip pull-down Wide-grip pull-down	Close-grip chin-up Wide-grip chin-up
BACK	Bent over dumbbell rows Bent over barbell rows	Cable rows One-arm rows
ABS	Crunches Abdominal curls Machine curls	Lying leg raises Hanging leg raises Knee raises
QUADS	Dumbbell squats Barbell squats	Leg extensions Machine leg presses
HAM-STRINGS	Lunges Leg curls	Straight-leg deadlifts
CALVES	Standing calf raises Seated calf raises	Machine calf raises Donkey calf raises

Some exercise options require specialized equipment found in a fitness club. Please seek a personal trainer for assistance.

GET MORE FREE

Stay highly motivated   Never stop learning

MAKE HEALTH THE FOUNDATION OF YOUR LIFE

Learn MORE about a

Healthy and Vibrant Life

right to your eMail inbox

Visit

WWW.BETTERBODYBETTERLIFE.COM

and click on **"I got the book, give me more!"**

Use code:
BBoffer

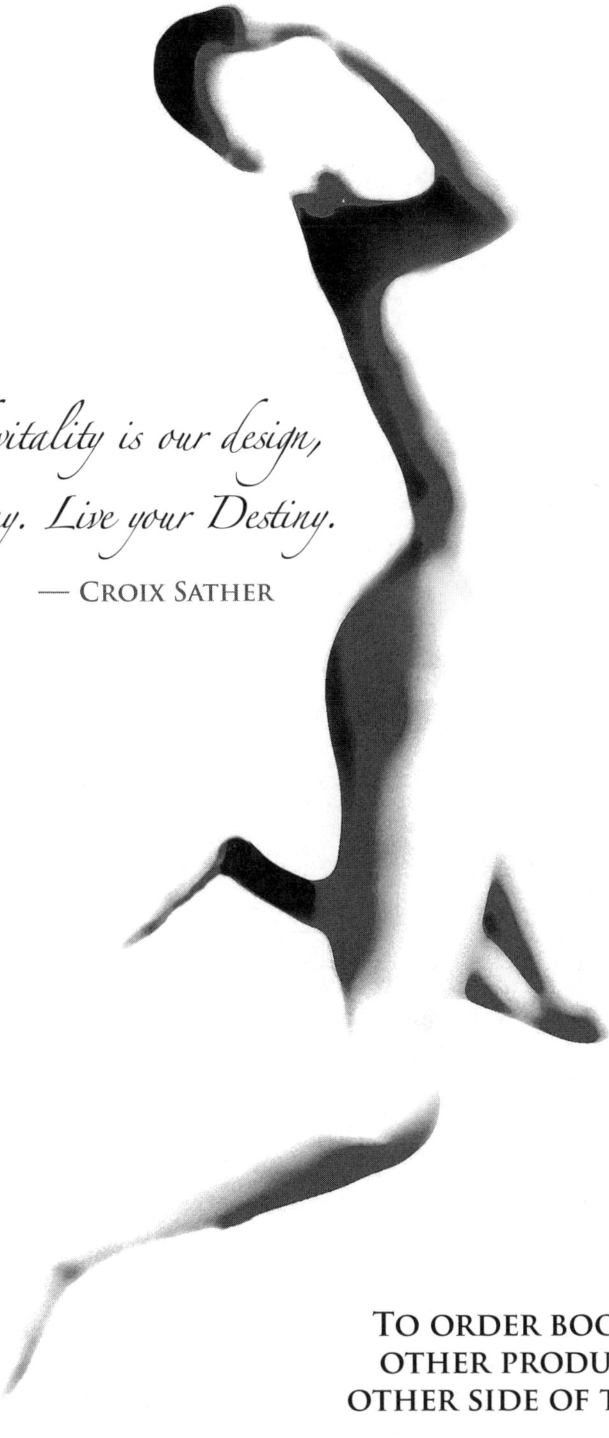

Health and vitality is our design,
it is our destiny. Live your Destiny.

— Croix Sather

To order books and other products see other side of this page

Give the gift of a BETTERBODY and a BETTERLIFE to friends and loved ones

Save MORE when you order online at
WWW.BETTERBODYBETTERLIFE.COM

☐ Yes, I want _______ copies of the BetterBody BetterLife book $19.99

☐ Yes, I want _______ copies of the BetterBody BetterLife Journal $15.99

☐ Yes, I want _______ copies of the BetterBody BetterLife DVD $19.99
Fit and Fabulous Body - Toning Edition

☐ Yes, I want _______ copies of the BetterBody BetterLife program that includes the book, journal, and fitness DVD at a huge discount for buying all three. ~~$55.97~~ retail — yours for only $44.99

Best deal
20% Discount for buying the complete program

☐ Yes, I want _______ copies of the abridged audiobook on CD $29.99
BetterBody BetterLife

Shipping and handling to anywhere in the continental USA add a flat rate of $4.50
Connecticut Residents please add 6% sales tax.

Check or money order for $ __________ is enclosed (payable to Renato Publishing)

Please charge my ☐ Visa ☐ Mastercard ☐ American Express

Card # ______________________________ Exp date __________

Name ____

Address ____

City/State/Zip _____________________________________

Phone ______________________ eMail ______________________

U.S. Mail orders: Renato Publishing - BB Order Department
PO Box 8834, New Fairfield, CT 06812

Telephone Orders: (866) 284-2213

eMail orders: orderservices@renatopublishing.com

Fax Orders: (203) 746-3747

Give the gift of a BETTERBODY and a BETTERLIFE
to friends and loved ones

Save MORE when you order online at
WWW.BETTERBODYBETTERLIFE.COM

☐ Yes, I want _______ copies of the BetterBody BetterLife book $19.99

☐ Yes, I want _______ copies of the BetterBody BetterLife Journal $15.99

☐ Yes, I want _______ copies of the BetterBody BetterLife DVD $19.99
Fit and Fabulous Body - Toning Edition

☐ Yes, I want _______ copies of the BetterBody BetterLife program that includes the book, journal, and fitness DVD at a huge discount for buying all three. ~~$55.97~~ retail — yours for only $44.99

Best deal 20% Discount for buying the complete program

☐ Yes, I want _______ copies of the abridged audiobook on CD $29.99
BetterBody BetterLife

Shipping and handling to anywhere in the continental USA add a flat rate of $4.50
Connecticut Residents please add 6% sales tax.

Check or money order for $ __________ is enclosed (payable to Renato Publishing)

Please charge my ☐ Visa ☐ Mastercard ☐ American Express

Card # ______________________________ Exp date __________

Name ____

Address ____

City/State/Zip_____________________________________

Phone__________________________eMail_________________________

U.S. Mail orders: Renato Publishing - BB Order Department
PO Box 8834, New Fairfield, CT 06812

Telephone Orders: (866) 284-2213

eMail orders: orderservices@renatopublishing.com

Fax Orders: (203) 746-3747